MW01098802

The

CHALLENGES

of

AGEING

*Reaching self-awareness,
acceptance & contentment*

MARIA CARMEN NAVARRO
NORMA MIRAFLOR

MEDIA MASTERS
SINGAPORE

The CHALLENGES *of* AGEING

© 2013 by Media Masters Pte Ltd

Published by:
Media Masters Pte Ltd
Newton Road P.O.Box 272
Singapore 912210

Email: mediamasters@singnet.com.sg
        mediam@bigpond.com

Website: www.mediamasters.com.sg

North American distribution:
Promontory Press
www.promontorypress.com

First published August 2013

Book design & layout: Demetrio Miraflor
Cover concept by courtesy: Bobot Reyes
Printed by: Mui Kee Press & Media 5 Pte Ltd, Singapore

No part of this publication may be reproduced in any form or by any means, electronic, mechanical, photocopying, recording or otherwise, without the prior consent of the publishers.

ISBN: 978-981-075-526-3

PREFACE

If you find, as you grow older, that the world is becoming more baffling – indeed, more disturbing – by the day, be assured you are not alone. Countless millions in your age bracket around our planet are experiencing similar feelings. In fact, they've been doing so for some years.

To suggest, then, that the publication of *The Challenges of Ageing* is timely, might well be an under-statement. After all, technical experts have, for over a decade now, been documenting the staggering impact population ageing is having on the very structure of human existence. It has been noted, for instance, that a large number of more developed countries – the United Kingdom, the European Community in general, the United States, Japan and Australia, among them – are all experiencing ageing population impacts never before encountered in human history.

A United Nations study on the subject estimates that the number of older persons worldwide tripled in a 50-year period to the year 2000. It will have more than tripled again by the year 2050. The impact on everyday living for older generations is massive. Unsurprisingly, an immense volume of related statistical reports on the subject is widely available. Decidedly less available, however, is down-to-earth information focussed on achieving rewarding ageing lives within these ever-intensifying environments.

Co-authors of *The Challenges of Ageing,* counselling psychologist, Maria Carmen Navarro, and novelist/historian, Norma Miraflor, have skilfully targeted this critical area of need. The result is a book for which there will surely be wide demand.

Far from being yet another statistical study, *The Challenges of Ageing* provides an absorbing account on coping with difficulties as the years roll on. It can be read, initially, for an overall appreciation of the ageing phenomenon. Thereafter it can be kept for valuable ready reference as life progresses.

CONTENTS

CHAPTER 1

WHERE HAVE THE YEARS GONE?

CHAPTER 2

STRATEGIES FOR MID-LIFE

CHAPTER 3

WORKING TOWARDS SELF-AWARENESS

CONTENTS

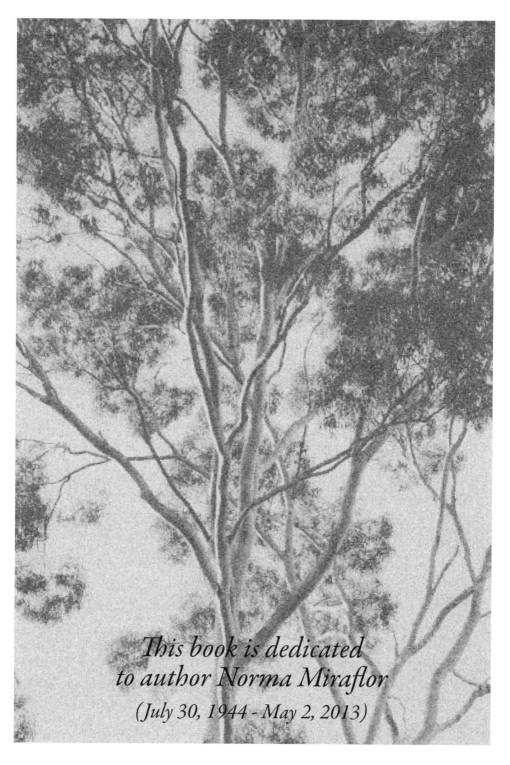

*This book is dedicated
to author Norma Miraflor*
(July 30, 1944 - May 2, 2013)

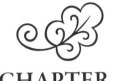

CHAPTER 1

WHERE HAVE THE YEARS GONE?
Youth escapes when we're looking the other way.

What have I been doing all these years?

Ageing springs its own surprises. We wake up one morning with a dull ache in the right knee. On an early evening, somebody hands us a brochure and the printed page is fuzzy; the letters overlap. The dentist thinks the last molar has to go. The six flights of stairs to have coffee with a confidant are no longer as enticing. When an acquaintance suggests a 10-hour journey by rail, we shoot back: are you kidding?

When it's inclement climate in the business community and people talk of redundancies, we immediately group ourselves with those who would be offered good-bye packages. Would there be life after early retirement?

Then there are the reports, the surveys and the statistics. They all talk of a greying world that has to contend with a variety of chronic illnesses. The topics are engaging, albeit sobering, because they are about *us*.

THE SURPRISING SHIFT

When did thoughts of ageing start cluttering your life?

If you gather a dozen people in a room and ask them that question, you would get a dozen different answers. Or you might end up with fifty replies because a few among the group would volunteer more than a single anecdote.

Conversations on ageing vary from person to person. There are people who sound old before they are 50 and there are those who manage to sparkle at 70. There are also those who give the impression they were born old and those who give no promise of growing up.

In the matter of that defining moment when one is jolted by the reality of ageing, here are some examples:

"After many years of resisting the yearly invitations, I finally decided to attend a school reunion. I had lost touch with most of my class and was aghast by the changes in all of us. I realised I had been too busy to notice even my own paunch. I came away totally devastated. I was 43."

"I used to enjoy trekking until I moved the family to the city and pursued a corporate life. One summer we rented a cottage and my two teenage sons and I went on daily walks. We were negotiating a hilly terrain one morning when I thought I was struggling to keep up with the boys. The heat and the steep craggy path did not trouble them at all. They were bantering and laughing all the way. Once or twice, one of them would ask, 'are you OK, Dad?'"

"I was 35 and my mother had just died. I had been working part-time because of her illness. My older brother asked me during the wake – 'so what are you planning to do now?' It dawned on me that both our parents were finally gone and that I was alone and I was no longer young. "

"One Christmas, an old schoolmate invited me to join his family during the holiday break. A tall good-looking girl opened the door. My friend introduced her as his eldest child, the one whose christening party I had attended. I was flummoxed."

"I went swimming with my nieces. I had always been proud of my figure. But on this particular afternoon I lingered by the life-size mirror in the changing room. The sight of cellulite – my own! – was a real downer."

"I was in a pub having a drink with an officemate. Out of the blue he asked, 'have you thought of what you might do when you retire?' "

"I went to one of our branch offices and the guy who met me at the station, he was in his late twenties, asked – 'would you like to rest first before going to the office, sir?' "

"My husband said, 'I think that dress would suit Tess better.' Tess is our daughter."

"I decided to have a child late in life. I was 39 and I was tired all the time throughout the pregnancy."

"I was watching my teenage daughter cycling away from the garden bench where my wife and I were seated. My wife said, 'soon she'll really be going away from us.' I started thinking of the legacy I could leave my only daughter."

"I was watching a politician peddling his election promises on TV when the thought sprung out: I was much older than the president of the United States of America!"

"I started looking furtively at my own body in department store changing rooms."

"The sales ladies began smiling indulgently when I chatted them up. In the good old days they exchanged jokes with me, or tried to anyhow."

"My father-in-law said – 'The two of us should now be able to understand each other.' "

"When trying to describe somebody, my niece said – 'She would be your age, not young but not so old.' "

"Armchairs became more attractive than bar stools."

"I found myself doing my sums more often, wondering whether my savings would be sufficient – what if I lived to, say, 90?"

"My passion for gardening began giving me aches and pains. My waist ached so much after a couple of hours' weeding."

"I started wondering whatever happened to my childhood friends."

"I realised I was sounding like my father."

Whatever the trigger, the ageing issue takes hold.

What happens?

The mind decides to "take stock" but the mind is also crammed with so many thoughts to make a proper job of it. How can we do a decent inventory of our lives thus far when we are also feeling rushed to complete countless disparate things before we are finally found decrepit and incapable? No wonder, the middle years are anxious, impatient and fretful years.

Our memory banks become erratic. Snippets from the past return. These are sharp and focused. The random flashbacks vary – snatches of conversation, bars from a half-remembered song, the image of a fruit basket or a rusty bicycle we hadn't thought of for years, fragments of a letter, somebody's voice. The thing is they come back for no rhyme or reason. You could be walking the dog in the park and – wham! – your mind's eye recalls a door, painted green, flanked by croton hedges, the house of your childhood.

A muddled sadness intrudes into our consciousness at odd moments. We feel an unexplained longing for things we can't either identify or describe.

Our conversations are often focused on health issues, the gaps between the attitudes of "this generation" and "our generation", absent friends and memories of "better times". Away from our peers, we start thinking we have become "invisible" in a crowd. When somebody forgets to call or a child does not visit as promised, we feel utterly rejected.

An expression – a sigh combining weariness, helplessness and resignation – often punctuates our pronouncements about the passage of time.

We linger over things. No more rushing to anything. We are no longer bothered if we haven't seen the latest blockbuster movie or read the number one bestseller or watched the most talked-about documentary of the month.

We come up with shorter lists. Our get-togethers become more informal and more intimate, reflecting discernment learned over the years. We are beginning to know whom we want to keep in our inner circle of friends. No more dissipating of energy.

We wonder whether the world is getting crazier or we are just getting more intolerant. We now feel entitled to say what we truly mean.

Names pop up in our minds – former classmates, former teachers, former neighbours, old acquaintances – and we wonder whatever happened to them.

Associations overlap. When we come across a familiar face, it takes longer for us to place it. We wonder – a playmate from childhood? A university acquaintance? A colleague from a previous job? A former neighbour?

We endeavour to reconcile the face we confront in the mirror with the clever, quick-witted and highly mobile self we've perceived in us for years.

A requirement for simplicity gets more resonance. There is a nagging sense of the need to let go. More and more we feel the requirement to de-clutter life, to clear spaces of superfluous items and the need for more time on our own. Instead of acquiring more possessions, we find it easier to give away keepsakes.

All of a sudden – for that's how it feels in the beginning – we get rooted to a spot with all the confused emotions that come with situations foisted on us.

Ageing is not our choice. It just happens to us. Sometimes, it brings with it a sense of relief that, now, we might be able to confront many issues with some degree of wisdom.

But we also realise that a few wonderful things are steadily slipping away or being drained from us – spontaneity, desire, ambition and the capacity to glory in the claim that we can burn our candle at both ends. We resent and mourn our losses.

The spectre of utter uselessness in the not-so-distant future proves alarming. The idea that we would, sooner than we expect it, be considered irrelevant, like a piece of old unwanted furniture, is enough for us to turn paranoid, impatient and cantankerous.

Ageing can be a fretful stage. But you have the choice to transform it to a worthwhile adventure.

"I was a 47-year-old banker," recalls Victor. "I was in what was referred to as middle management. When the cost-cutting exercise started in our bank, I hadn't expected the panic that set in. I had sleepless nights. I walked around the block wondering what would happen if I got retrenched. My wife and I were then paying a mortgage and had two boys still at school. Fortunately, I was spared the axe. But I learned from that horrible time. I realised we did not have to live in a five-bedroom house. We did not have to think of overseas holidays as a must just because our friends were flying everywhere. We sold our house, paid off the mortgage and placed the spare cash in a term deposit.

I also thought of what I could do when my banking life was over. I have always been interested in gardening and one of my sons suggested we could start a small gardening maintenance business. In the beginning it was a weekend thing but it soon started to roll into a constant money-making venture. Neither of my sons was academically inclined and by the time the older one was in Year 12, we had decided to go into partnership full time. My younger son announced he would get into the tiling trade. When I turned 50, I had had enough of working at a desk and wearing a tie. I'm 56 now and glad I got a wake-up call early. I'm not a rich man but I can sleep soundly and start the day with no fear of getting the sack. I must say that having a good cooperative family helps a lot."

There are the more problematic instances when health issues force us to look closer at our lives and consider how we would conduct ourselves if we were granted more time on this planet.

Bronte, a 65 year-old graphic designer, reminisces about lying in a hospital bed when she was 49 years old. She had had a radical mastectomy and despaired at the thought that she would never see 50.

"It was a life-changing period," Bronte writes. "My world had turned upside down. I was lucky I had a good marriage. My husband and I journeyed through the diets, the meditation, the radiotherapy sessions and the clinical depression that seemed to be interminable. I was like a changed person for a few years after the mastectomy. Then one day I found myself laughing again, as in the old days.

"But something had definitely changed. I became more focused on the present. I now give whatever it is I'm doing my full attention, whether it is drawing a butterfly or draining pasta or playing with my grandchildren. To this day, after 16 years, I don't make long-range plans. You may call it superstition. I don't care what it is. I just can't say I'm saving to holiday in Acapulco in two or three years. Suffice that I am in this moment and I am not troubled by envy or greed or past grudges."

The dampening effects of ageing may at times be triggered by minor, even trivial, episodes. Depending on our values, we could be deeply affected by the discovery of a few grey locks or the loosening of skin or the possibility of wearing dentures.

Our earlier training and the nature of our character, in turn, determine our reactions to the obvious and undeniable signs that we are no longer the young people who once thought they were immortal.

WE GET TOO BUSY TO REMEMBER

The story is the same for everybody. Childhood is too brief and before we know it people are telling us to remember our age – we have turned into adults with responsibilities!

Adulthood comes with the right we had dreamed of as children – the freedom to choose what to do with our lives. Our world gets peopled with friends and acquaintances who share the same interests and prejudices. We put in extra hours to advance in our careers. We schedule trips to destinations ostensibly to broaden our minds. We enjoy being pushed to the limit of our capabilities and like saying that we thrive on challenges. We even enjoy the criticism that we have little time for our families – inferring that we are kept preoccupied by something bigger and more important. After all, we explain, our career or our job is the very thing that puts food on the table, pays for the car, educates the children and meets the insurance premiums.

We become serious people with big objectives. We refine our tastes and surround ourselves with proof of success. It pleases us when others comment on the fact that "we have arrived". We accumulate things and surround ourselves with possessions.

As the years fly, the line between our needs and our wants gets totally blurred. We become obsessed with "bettering ourselves" which we measure in the largeness of our houses and the sheen of our cars. This burgeoning period appears to go on and on.

We forget to worry about having to maintain the momentum of all the headiness. We start to think that we are indeed luckier than most. This lasts until the trimmings begin losing their allure. Until we realise the children are grown and have begun talking about knowing how to lead their lives. Until it is no longer fun to claim that we like burning the candle at both ends. Until a pinched nerve unnerves us.

When Arthur, now 62, became Chief Operations Officer (COO) of a multi-national corporation in his mid-40s, he considered his achievement as one forged by luck. He was aware of his quick mind, his competence and his devotion to work. But he also knew he had competed for the post against four others who were as bright and as efficient as he was. So he thought that of the five of them, he had more luck.

The company shares allotted to him yearly with the parallel rise of their worth on the stock market somehow loosened Arthur's grip on reality. What made him buy a Jaguar after many years of being content with a trusted, reliable nondescript five-year-old saloon car? What made him dissatisfied with the terrace house he had lived in for the better part of 10 years? Why did he suddenly want to play golf and be a member of exclusive clubs?

Simply, Arthur forgot that he wouldn't be COO forever and that the share market was as volatile as his marriage. In the market crash of 1987, Arthur's shares were reduced to zilch; worse, because he had borrowed on margins, he owed money. While he needed to remain COO, he found it difficult to get going in the mornings because he always woke up remembering he had a mortgage, a car loan and a bag of shares that, in the meantime, were worthless. He also had to contend with an angry wife. Daily, she reminded him that she was against the Jaguar, against the blasted new house and against the pretentious golf club. She said he had changed and not for the better; she declared the desire to leave him.

The upshot was a divorce, a return to a smaller car and a contraction to a private but minuscule flat because his now ex-wife and their three children were deemed more deserving of a terrace house. Arthur remained COO for another two years but in that time he became acutely aware that he was no longer young.

"Good fortune can make you lose track of the basic things," Arthur notes. "Turning 50 did not worry me at all because I was driving a Jag and I could buy the champagne that flowed so freely. For a while I thought the gravy train would go on rolling. Well, it didn't. When it stopped I became aware I was ageing and had to adapt to the changing circumstances. I was depressed for a long time."

Similarly, Owen, 60 and Leila, 62, had always wanted a Range Rover and on a bright spring morning they trundled off to acquire the car of their dreams. But with the gleaming British racing green vehicle parked in the carport, Leila's nerve wobbled.

"Perhaps we got carried away," Leila confides. "I ended up thinking we had splurged good money on something that was, after all, only a whim. To be honest, Owen was probably swayed by my rhapsodizing about wishing to drive a Range Rover for years and wanted to please me. When we finally got it, I realised I'd truly desired it only in the earlier years when I imagined driving a Range Rover with the children singing in the back seat. But the children had left home by the time we bought it."

Our genuine appreciation for objects is intertwined with the more important things in our lives. Without the association with those meaningful aspects, objects remain objects, things are just things – inanimate items we can use for convenience or move around and group and re-group until we tire of them. *Possessions assume significance only if they are made to represent something that holds meaning for us.*

We can produce a chronicle of incidents duplicating Owen and Leila's experience with their dream car. Somewhere along the line we get it into our heads that *something* will make us happy. Whatever it is, the longing seeps deep into our consciousness where it sits and becomes part of our life story.

Few among us make the effort to examine this specific want and dislodge it if it no longer tallies with our current reality. So for years and years we remain vaguely believing we want a cellar or a large patio or special suitcases. When we finally get what we desire – cellar or patio or suitcases – we see that we had wanted the cellar in the years when we regularly gathered friends to sample our latest wine discoveries. Or we had longed for a large patio because the man of the house was a whiz at barbecues. Or we desired beautiful luggage because we were then tireless corporate warriors.

Finally getting *what we've always wanted* is often not aligned with our present reality. For instance, most of our fellow wine-lovers who enjoyed our wine samplings may have drastically modified their drinking habits. Or the patio would be irrelevant because the barbecue get-togethers stopped when the beloved chef died five years ago. Or the impressive suitcases would be superfluous because we have opted for early retirement.

In all these examples possession proves disappointing because it has no relevance to the present. The reason behind the requirement at the time the yearning for it was hatched no longer exists.

The passage of time is a fact of life we take for granted until it is driven home by realities that affect us personally. In Leila's case, ageing was underlined by the discovery that her wish for the Range Rover was woven with the pleasure she got from the songs her children sang together as she drove them from place to place. It is with some melancholy that she views the dream car. It is a constant reminder that her children, now adults with lives of their own, would never again serve as her backseat choir.

An obvious decline in energy is another reality the ageing confront. Sluggishness sets in. Regular rest periods become more attractive. The to-do list gets shorter.

A 69-year old retired stockbroker recalls: "My wife and I were in Tuscany when I found myself thinking that I much preferred to linger in the courtyard of this quaint hotel to joining the other tourists on the bus. I was in my late 50s then. Before a trip, my wife and I usually prepared a list of things we would like to do together and another list to accommodate our separate interests. That particular time in Tuscany, however, I was dragging myself through the first list and ignoring the second one completely. One afternoon my wife came back from one of her market tours and found me reading on the balcony of our room. She sat opposite me and sighed. 'How's the market?' I asked. She was looking wistfully at the hanging baskets of geraniums above her. 'I just got tired,' she said. I tapped her hand and said, 'same here'. We then decided the yearly long trips were getting us down and that we'd forgotten we were not as young as we used to be. In our 30s, the success of a trip was measured in the number of monuments we saw. We now take short trips. We still go to Europe, but once every three or four years."

Pacing ourselves is another adjustment to make. Unlike the retired stockbroker we may find it difficult to admit to our diminishing strengths and get into a denial mode. Some are caught up in denial for a long time. We could keep on hopping on tour buses and working our way through lists of where to go or what to do. In so doing we run the risk of losing what used to be genuine interest and having it replaced by the empty boast that things remain unchanged. Examined closely, we indeed manage but we are changed – half the time we are cross with peddlers who pester us with their goods. Incompetent guides bother us. We look forward to our hotel rooms, for the quietness there and the opportunity to put our feet up.

Michael, 64, is a year away from retirement. For most of his life he had crammed his non-working schedule with the interests that made the stresses of corporate life bearable. He read voraciously, went to the cinema regularly, visited galleries where friends were exhibiting their works and was an enthusiastic theatregoer.

"No longer," Michael says. "I used to rush out and get a copy of the latest best-seller and I had to see whether the reviews were right about a movie or a concert or a play. I was always part of the queue. These days I don't feel the need to rush for anything. I am still interested in reading and the movies and the theatre but I'm not bothered by the thought that I might be missing out on something. I can read today's bestseller next year or the year after next. It doesn't matter. You can say I have stopped being frantic to be among the first to know about something. I am aware this is part of ageing and I don't mind it, not at all. In fact, I'm grateful I've stopped being frenetic about a lot of things."

NOSTALGIA SETS IN

We recall sadly how we used to blithely negotiate countless flights of stairs, skipping up steps, three at a time. The distance between our fast and slower selves is more than a dispiriting mile. In looking back to examine the yawning gulf we confront a great number of realities – we are not just walking slower and covering shorter distances but our social network has likewise contracted with the departures or defections of friends. Should we still dare discuss career possibilities at this point? More and more we convince ourselves to be extra cautious about major risks, whether they be in financial investments or in complex travel plans.

A father confides in an email to his son: "Your Uncle Fred and I were just on Skype and he was asking, 'hey, what happened to us? We used to talk about our sexual exploits, the true ones and the imagined ones. Listen to us now, Pete,' he said. 'We are talking about aches and prescriptions, discussing our blood pressure and comparing cholesterol readings. We used to compete over the ladies. Now it's a contest of who has more health issues.' Now, my dear son, don't chuckle so much. Your day will come before you know it. What I'm trying to say is don't be like your dad a hundred per cent. Watch the frequency of the beer mugs, etc. etc."

We are left wondering where the years have gone. And what have we been up to all this time? Where is the sprightly 20-year-old who could dance all night, the dismissive one who believed her 45-year-old aunt was out of touch and irrelevant? Where is the 25-year-old impertinently carefree person who was convinced he would conquer the world?

Here's a sample email from one (used to be) indefatigable cartoonist to another (used to be) fire-in-the-belly type journalist: "Ok, let's meet at Jo's. Easier to park and no stairs to climb. 4.30pm. No problem; I can witness the docs. Then why don't we have coffee? Oh how our drinking habits have changed!"

Alison, a 52-year-old chiropractor volunteers: "I had a very successful practice. Then, in my mid-40s it became clear to me that I could not go on filling my appointment book five days in a row. I had been doing it for a while and there came a point I was too tired to meet friends on the weekend. I suppose you reach a junction when you make choices. I don't like being too tired to laugh. "

VIEWING THE BALANCE SHEET

In her book *Growing Old, A Journey of Self-Discovery*, D. Quinodoz (translation by D. Alcorn, 2010, East Sussex, UK, Routledge), asserts the conceptual definition of ageing deals with three patterns – normal, optimal and pathological.

- Normal (or usual) ageing – refers to a process dominant within a society for persons who are not suffering from a manifest illness. It is ageing without biological or mental pathology. The usual aches and pains occur and a number of complaints surface with the deterioration of physical strengths. Old age may even be visited by fragility or failing health. But, on the whole, life proceeds with a certain calm and lucidity. Most of us would fall under this category.

- Optimal or successful ageing – growing old with the support of development-enhancing and age-friendly environmental conditions. This is a kind of utopia where a developed society grants the ageing and the aged the same importance granted to the young and those who are in the pinnacle of their earning or productive powers. This is the kind of ageing enjoyed by those who have applied strategies required to meet the demands of every developmental stage.

- Pathological ageing – where the subject undergoes syndromes of illness and the ageing process is determined by the study of the cause of disease. Continuing denial and constant refusal to accept past and present realities result in more mistakes, more regrets and additional bitterness. In turn, these can often trigger various undiagnosed neuroses. People whose ageing is determined by medical etiology (the study of the cause of disease) and syndromes of illness belong to this group along side dementia or Alzheimer sufferers.

The basic dynamics of later life reflect two subtle but profound shifts. Firstly, there is a changing balance between gains and losses. Secondly, there occurs an increasing investment of the individual's reserve capacity towards maintenance functions, rather than growth.

Of course we mourn the loss of our unflappable, tireless selves. This is a natural phase that should run its course. Only after we have accepted that we are no longer young can we truly move on to the next stages of our lives.

What is this period of mourning like? We exchange stories of how we used to be dauntless and how we thought we were probably the epicentres of the universe. At the same time, we listen to the consolation prizes that come with seniority – we can now be more articulate; we are more discerning; we can keep our emotions in check and look after ourselves; we are clear with the choices we make and we are now able to regulate and control our lives.

There is no time limit to this phase. Its conclusion is determined by our varying dispositions. There are people who get reconciled to the realities of ageing faster and better than others. There are those who wish to hold back the onslaught of time and look to reprieve by undergoing cosmetic surgery, blundering into random love affairs and spending hours making up for what was missed during the earlier years, whether it is through dancing all night or partying endlessly or travelling constantly.

Larry's parents divorced when Larry was 36. His mother was 56. Larry says, "My mother just went berserk. She was booking flights right, left and centre. She went on three long-haul trips in one year. I would call her up and she'd say, 'Oh I'm off to Czechoslovakia' or Andorra or Bhutan. Or she would be buying so many concert subscriptions and go out even when she was feeling unwell.

"I know she was making up for the years when she merely tagged along and was virtually my dad's shadow. But I also thought it was my duty to tell her to take it easy. She would get upset and say she wasn't willing to postpone doing things for herself and get on a rant about my dad being a control freak and how I was beginning to sound like him. I suppose that was the start of the small rift between us. They have been divorced four years now and I'm a 40-year-old optometrist with a mother who's still booking flights and going to concerts as if there was no tomorrow."

There is no substitute for youth, say the gurus, but there's nothing like wisdom. The question is, how do we arrive at this wisdom that helps us navigate the choppy waters of ageing so that we can divest ourselves of the residues of rancour and arrive at our desired destination – a quiet, peaceful, and gracious old age?

The world is ever changing and unless we accept that we have to change, we will find it difficult to adapt to our altering surroundings.

A 74-year-old historian notes: "As a 10-year-old boy I used to spend my school holidays in Perth. I vividly remember the woman whose house we used to stay in. She liked wearing white. She also took pleasure in whingeing. Part of the time I was amused because she was complaining about things I knew, like the telephone. She didn't like it because she said it stopped people from visiting or writing letters to one another; now they were just yakking on the telephone. But most of the time she directed her tirades at changing modes of travel. She liked travelling by sea. She hated cars. At the dinner table she talked about how she found the world so confounding. She complained about the drop in standards in every aspect of life. She didn't like anything about the world and was always talking about how things were much nicer and better when she was younger. I listened to all that and thought, what a strange person. I was 10 and, unlike her, I found my surroundings exciting and promising. How could she be such a grouch? I remember her because my life has reached a point when not much of my surroundings make much sense to me."

A Later-life Balance Sheet: losses & gains

The losses

Physical strengths – A "slowing down" which is not something we arrive at by choice. Our bodies tell us when we have to stop and sit back so we may re-group. The physical loads we could handle easily a decade ago assume the proportions of monumental burdens to be taken "little by little" and between reasonable intervals. Refusals to listen to our bodies result in ill health. People who don't indulge in constant conversations with their bodies are more prone to feel out-of sorts, catch colds and be down with the 'flu more often than those who rest when they feel fatigue setting in.

"The older one gets," observes Nelly, 53, "the bigger handbag you need. You require space for your reading glasses, your looking glasses and your sunglasses. There's got to be a compartment for your little prescription bottles. Your wallet has to be organised or you'll end up taking forever in sorting out the coins while the whole room waits. The little paperback or your son's Kindle should be in your bag too because, as your son would remind you, you could very well leave it in the restaurant loo."

"I'm hard of hearing in my left ear," chips in Amelia, 67, "and have to ask people to sit on my right. These days, I miss half the conversation at a long table. Pretty soon I have to get a hearing aid, but I remember how my mother used to be upset with hers. She claimed it didn't do much good, only magnified background noises and filled her head with rage."

Cognitive processing – The older we get the longer we take responding to questions and the more frequent the need to be reminded about things. We feel the requirement to sift carefully through ideas presented before forming an opinion and voicing it. Complex impressions take time to register and leave us more often hemming and hawing.

Frank, 46, points to anxiety over the correctness of his responses. "It wasn't like this in my early 30s. Then I was quick with my replies and retorts. But these days I find myself weighing the pros and cons of my reactions to ideas before sharing them. I think as we grow older we become aware that we may not really know that much about anything so we run things through our minds repeatedly until they are crystal clear to us."

Chris, 59, keeps a diary. Self-employed, he does not have an assistant to remind him of his schedule. "I had no problem until I got into my early 50s. My memory was brilliant. I could remember names, addresses and telephone numbers. Then, one fine day, I turned into this stranger who forgot that he had arranged to meet a pal in the pub. So I started to keep a diary and now check it every night so I don't miss appointments. I don't want to be thought of as slackening in my old age. I think we get bombarded by too much information, layer upon layer of useless trivia, and this has affected our working memory. These days I try to avoid too much TV and I'm not a Google fiend."

Income – Unless we have built a business empire and started a private dynasty of CEOs, ageing sees a gradual and continuing diminution of our earning capacities. We may wish to go on working at the same job we have had for years but our age or our diminished energies or even the daily commute may decide against it. We could decide to work part-time but even this might prove too much after a while.

Attitude towards risk-taking – We get less adventurous as we age. The things that we dismiss as "part of the franchise" when we are young tend to get magnified. The possibility of falling ill or losing our luggage or missing our connecting flight or our cousin failing to be at the airport when we arrive assume frightful proportions that make us travel less and less.

In our youth, we found it amusing when we were advised about considering "rainy days". How tedious such reminders were! But something happened along the way and rainy day thoughts have become our reality. They make us think twice, many times, before embarking on projects. We consider so many "what ifs", with a tendency to look at the downside. Our reactions are not as fast; our decisions are delayed. We become too cautious.

We become very involved in reviewing our savings and investments. What we used to consider as sufficient now appears inadequate in the light of global changes and our keener awareness of the likely possibility of illness or our living to a great age.

We become more concerned over where the trajectories of our emotional decisions might lead us. Embarking on new relationships becomes doubly hard. A 45-year-old contemplating marriage for the first time finds it more exercising to reach a decision than a man in his late 20s because he no longer enjoys the excuse of youth and inexperience. It is taken for granted that, at a certain stage of our lives, we have learned from our mistakes and therefore should know better.

Declines in vision and hearing – More than thinning hair that most people can blame on genes or a nutritional deficiency, detached retina or hearing aids that don't work make ageing doubly challenging for the afflicted.

George, a widower at 51, was at a cocktail party where he got very attracted to an elegant woman named Lisa. As the evening deepened, the din of background noise became oppressive and his hearing aid failed him utterly. But George hung on, gripping his gin and tonic valiantly as Lisa chatted away beside him. He nodded and smiled, smiled and nodded. The next day, George's officemate, who witnessed the entire episode, dropped by and chided: "Lisa thinks you're weird. She says you would not answer the simplest questions. Better call her up and tell her you're deaf." They both laughed but George was left feeling despondent. What to do now? What if he finds it difficult to hear her again? Would Lisa care to go out with someone who was hard of hearing?

In another case, the eye doctors advised Dan to minimise his reading, TV viewing and Internet activity. This irked him but what he really minded was the fact that he could no longer enjoy the brilliance of things around him. His failing vision dulled the world for him and he mourned this because he was a very visual person. Most of his life Dan had congratulated himself for being able to name hues and shades of objects – burnt sienna, old rose, ochre. It therefore mattered a lot to him that teal now appeared to be a messy blob that was neither green nor blue.

Visual or hearing impairment severely affects a person's sense of independence. The news that one should stop driving a car or the requirement for a companion on outings is naturally met with resistance and can cause severe depression.

A strong sense of isolation and vulnerability – The decline in physical powers and the thinning circle of trusted friends could make us feel all alone. Naturally we insist on sticking to our life-long image of ourselves – independent, self-sufficient, strong – and therefore hedge on calling trusted parties who would help us remain active participants of society. This could be our ultimate undoing. Misplaced pride could expose us to the manipulative ways of people who would sense our need to belong and take advantage of our weakened emotional state.

Social network – For the most part of our productive years, busy schedules and time constraints make us socialise with people with whom we work closely and do business. Convenience makes us believe they are our friends. For a very long while, we lose touch with the good friends of our youth whose company we'd wished to keep. As ageing sets in and our circumstances change, we sort out priorities. The meaning of friendship becomes important again. It is a sad reality of ageing that when we finally get around to reaching out to old friends, very few can be found. Many may have moved to other cities or even countries; a few may have died and many more simply cannot be tracked down.

Ageing is the time when the quality of one's remaining friendships must be enhanced.

Roles – We must always allow for change. As we age, so do our circumstances and we must be prepared to accept the adjustments necessary to make the present less stressful. Our children grow up and we have to let go. We cannot insist on them following our suggestions on how they should conduct their lives – often we base our advice only on what makes **us** happy.

We should not be aggrieved by our shrinking roles in the world

– hopefully we'd done our fair share of productive, if frantic, living. We should be glad all the loving and losing, the choosing and regretting, the taking a chance and winning – happened to us. We should now have the grace to sit back and watch others – people younger than we are – wear themselves out.

The gains

Verbal skills for needs and requirements – Children are often asked: *what exactly do you mean?* In our youth, conflicting emotions made it hard to put our expectations in a nutshell. Sometimes, we held back, afraid to displease or disappoint. As we grew older, our hopes were clarified and our long lists of wishes got shortened. We felt the requirement to be heard and given the chance to work towards our objectives.

Fruitful ageing happens when people are able to make use of this capacity to voice their true feelings.

Social discernment – Ageing puts great emphasis on the quality, not the quantity, of friendships and associations. It is very comforting to reach a stage when one is accepted for what one is and accepts others in the same vein.

Emotional balance and self-regulation – As we grow older, the need to be centred is addressed more assiduously. We acknowledge that while we hold very strong emotions about many issues, so do others and it's proof of maturity when we acknowledge the validity of other views. We no longer need a parent or a boyfriend or a wife to remind us to behave well or to stop being rude. We can be our own cops.

Clarity of values – Ageing calls for a review of our attitudes towards many issues. We analyse how they rank in importance – family, friendship, work and money. If we have to, we summon the courage to adapt or adjust. Once our values are clear to us, they will be evident to those who share our environment. The clarity of our values enables us to set our boundaries, making it easier for others to see how much space we would be willing to share. Saying no or working out a reasonable compromise is not difficult if we are sure of our priorities.

Family and role choices – We are able to decide for ourselves the part we wish to play in the changed circumstances. We stop cajoling or patronising family members. We choose to avoid emotional blackmail. We are now adults, like our parents and our older siblings and we should talk to one another as adults respecting one another. This is a true plus factor in successful ageing. No more mind games.

Personality complexity – We are able to examine our motives and try to examine what drives others. We see the need for compassion and empathy. We are less dismissive but neither do we allow ourselves to be overwhelmed by somebody else's perceptions.

A balanced sense of entitlement – We acknowledge that we are not the epicentre of the universe and other people, no matter how dear or close they are to us – have the right to their own time and interests.

A healthy sense of attachment to people and possessions – We finally learn that in order to keep relationships we shouldn't throttle the objects of our affection. Similarly, we refuse to be held hostage by material possessions.

Expertise and wisdom – Ageing should make us see the world with an openness learned through a lifetime of both happiness and heartbreak. We should now be able to view it with knowing eyes.

CHAPTER 2

STRATEGIES FOR MID-LIFE

This is in reply to the thousands who ask: I'm healthy but how come I've ended up feeling like 90 years old when I get up in the morning? I know I've got unresolved issues and will address them in time. But right now I have to earn a living and I'm too busy. Are there ways of making the present less of a load?

Everyone desires longevity but nobody wants to age. This is one of the puzzling ironies of life.

Conveniently, we take shelter under the umbrella of middle age. Of course the middle years are a fretful, challenging and testing time. We still have jobs to keep and rise with a heavy heart each morning to wear our social masks. It is trying and tiring to feel that a great part of our lives may have been spent toiling at things we hardly enjoyed or dealing with people we couldn't care less about.

It is around this time that many aspects of our lives are subjected to much conjecture and censure – our relationships, our parenting skills, our standing in the community and our associations with colleagues at work. Major changes could also occur during these years, like moves to another state or country due to work, or even a decision to migrate. These could test our competence and endurance.

But in terms of chronological age, mid-life gives some comfort to those who fear old age. Psychologically, there is still a big slice of the future ahead – there's still time on one's side. A great number of people seek to extend this refuge for as long as possible, believing and declaring themselves middle-aged at 50. Why so? We wish to postpone the acceptance of full-on ageing. The self-deception is helped if one could refer to decrepit parents and assorted hobbling relations. One could still talk about the transition to old age, a bridge to the future and adjustments to make.

Of course mid-life has its complications but for most of us being "middle-aged" is better than being "aged". No matter that we sometimes wake up feeling like 90 years old – and this need not happen.

HOW WELL DO YOU KNOW YOUR BODY?

While physical deterioration occurs naturally with ageing, we can arrest the slide and enable the body to enjoy a reprieve. Coupled with a philosophical attitude towards the advancing years, we may yet achieve optimal ageing.

Had you listened to your high school teacher and retained those nuggets of information he or she had struggled to make you hear, you would have paid more attention to how your body functions and addressed its specific needs accordingly.

You would not be taking up brisk walking only at 46 because there's this recurring pain in your joints. Caring for your bones would have started long before your 20s when, according to rheumatology specialists, bone-building cells (osteoblasts) are no longer as active and rapid in replacing broken-down old bones as they do in children.

It is amusing how men and women go through their lives preoccupied with thoughts of baldness or sagging breasts when they should really be more interested in the loss of neurons (the nerve cells that affect brain function), the balance of unfriendly and friendly bacteria in the gut (a good balance equals a good digestive system), the lessening of elasticity in blood vessels (they determine the quality of blood circulation around the body) and the steady reduction in the number of nephrons (the units used as filters that rid the bloodstream of waste).

The brain is arguably the part of the body that determines our ultimate approach to the ageing issue. Left idle and alone, it could result in various neuroses and even pathological ageing.

Those of us who insist on looking at the man with the Rolls Royce – and whinge about an uneven playing field – should take heart: as a general rule, we all start with 100 billion nerve cells (neurons) in the brain. This neuron bank begins getting depleted when we are in our 20s. In our middle years we can be losing as much as 10,000 neurons a day. Our memory and our capacity to reason are invariably affected by these daily losses. In certain cases, even balance or coordination can show signs of wear and tear.

So the brain has to be exercised and nourished from childhood. Making children understand the tales read to them at bedtime is important. The requirement that the young, aged 10 or 11, explain what they really mean when they talk to adults has similar value. The expectations that the children should understand signs, books, pictures, etc, are all firmly based concepts.

As we grow older, mental calisthenics become even more important. The brain needs to be regularly exercised and tested. The 70-year-old guy engrossed in a crossword puzzle, the 64-year-old woman learning French and the 58-year-old divorcee who has taken up piano lessons for the first time in her life are doing themselves a greater favour than the 45-year-old who believes that the anxiety accompanying ageing would be alleviated by a cosmetic surgeon.

If we had been aware that lung capacity gradually and steadily decreases from our 20s, we would perhaps not have smoked at all and instead got more interested earlier in the fight for a much cleaner environment.

Even if negative genetic considerations are taken into account, there's always the hope that the utmost care and attention we give our brains, our guts, our bones, our lungs, our hearts, our livers and our kidneys might just carry us through our ageing years with less grief than our predecessors faced.

Parents should understand how their children's knowledge and care of the body will give them a decided advantage in life. This is very important. The young need to be encouraged to look after themselves and told why they have to eat their vegetables and do their physical exercises and brush their teeth. Just saying, 'do this and do that because I told you so' has never worked and never will.

The lessons of early life are often met with resistance because they are commandments delivered without accompanying incentives and clarification.

Those of us who did not enjoy an enlightened childhood could still catch up by discovering, with the help of our GPs and clinicians, how to stem the rapid loss of neurons, osteoblasts and whatever else that enable us to function.

TYPES OF AGEING

There are different types of ageing – chronological, emotional and psychological. Most of us tend to focus on numbers and surface appearances, neglecting to take into account that emotional and psychological issues play a great part in why some people manage to take ageing in their stride, while others appear deeply troubled by it.

The need to survive in a highly competitive world and the requirement to abide by social norms make it instinctive for most people to hide their true feelings. A person may smile out of politeness when he could be actually seething inside. To save his job or to keep the peace at home, he may have to regularly wear a social mask. The cumulative effect of this repeated disharmony between the person's outer and inner selves results in considerable disquiet.

After years and years of following the dictates of society and wearing social masks, many people still suffer in silence, hedge at discussing their innermost thoughts and baulk at the idea of counselling.

Mid-life often gets beset by the subconscious desire for the chronological, emotional and psychological phases of ageing to mesh, signifying the individual's liberation from past developmental traps.

The "mid-life crises" people undergo are actual manifestations of their desire for such liberation. They are "cries for help" from those who feel fragmented and desire to be "whole" again. Of course, in so many instances, efforts have backfired and the subjects concerned end up with more emotional problems to sort out. People have walked out of good jobs; withdrawn men suddenly take to leather jackets and sports cars; housewives talk endlessly about "flings" at coffee mornings and plan dream trips abroad; husbands take their secretaries to mountain retreats and, without warning, a businessman could give away his worldly goods to least likely recipients.

Something triggers the desire for self-integration and the "explosion" could be personally mismanaged.

The "trigger" digs deeper during mid-life and it makes the period truly challenging. The subconscious desire to harmonise one's personality and organise it into a whole person (ego integration) is always confronted by the innate resistance to recognise repressed impulses and the need finally to do away with defence mechanisms (ego resistance).

Isobel, 39, confides: "My insomnia is getting worse and I get up in the morning feeling exhausted. My GP suggests it may have something to do with my wish to resume my postgraduate studies in Linguistics that were put on hold when my son was born six years ago. Something stops me from bringing it up with my husband. Honestly, I don't know how he'd react. I find so many excuses to postpone bringing it up. Meanwhile, I feel I'm not making the most of my life."

You may have wondered about those people unable to settle in dream jobs, or about those who could never land the ideal holiday, or men and women who could never find anything good to say about nearly everything.

The reason is not the absence of dream jobs or the lack of excellent destinations or the darkness of the universe. The re-examination of the world should begin with the person complaining about the gloom. How genuine is his/her desire for authenticity, for a better life, and for harmony? How self-aware is this person?

It is what this chapter is all about.

THE INNER SELF

Many people confront ageing with a renewed concern for their health. This should be commended. As is often said, better late than never. Regular trips to the gym, walking briskly, swimming laps, cycling, vitamin supplements and various antioxidants are added to the usual regimen of rushing to work and partying. Diets are revised to include more fruit and vegetables. Early to bed, early to rise is taken more seriously. The cocktail circuit assumes a back seat to quieter meals with the dear and near. Alcohol is no longer a consolation. Moderation becomes a mantra.

THERE ARE TOXINS OTHER THAN FAT DEPOSITS

Life is a journey with its many roads, intersections, stops and junctions. Life is also about choices. You and I have the right to go down a certain path and travel the way we wish. We can pursue long routes or opt for short cuts. We can run or dawdle; rush or take occasional pauses.

We will have to travel in all weathers. There will be storms, dips and hurdles. Some of the passions we'll pour our hearts into may fail to register. But there will also be days in the sun, feasts and, hopefully, a fair amount of fun and laughter.

The issue of ageing becomes paramount when we perceive that we have covered a considerable distance. As earlier stated, this perception often occurs with a suddenness that startles us. We have been functioning well and doing much, then one day it hits us – we don't get the same buzz we used to get from things. As somebody said a long time ago: middle age is when work is a lot less fun and fun is a lot more work.

Middle-aged, we begin examining our lives. What have we contributed to the world? Is there anything we can point out and say, with some satisfaction, *I did that*? What are we here for?

Nobody really feels cut out for the challenges of mid-life and ageing. Nobody is really *that* prepared for old age.

Nevertheless, we would want the journey to be well worth the effort. Regardless of gender and temperament, we would want to look back on something meaningful and significant.

At the crossroads, we would want it said that the years have not been wasted – that, by and large, it has been a worthwhile journey. In the final reckoning, regardless of the approaches and the choices made, nobody would ever want to review a wasteland.

So you may have rid your body of toxins but you still feel this heaviness.

Have you started examining your thoughts?

How big are the grudges you have kept locked up for years?

How much emotional baggage do you carry?

Ageing is more than just thinning of bones, sagging mouths or aching joints. The late eminent Hungarian endocrinologist, Dr Hans Selye – he coined the term "stress" and founded the International Institute of Stress – defined ageing as the sum total of all the scars and tensions of life. He went further and reminded us that the scars and wrinkles of ageing are often not just physical but in the medical sense, chemical and mental. It is this "internal stress" that brings about heaviness in the heart and troubled sleep.

If only we could expel both the physical and mental toxins that make us stay awake in the wee small hours, angry or eaten up by guilt or regrets!

The quality of the body-mind connection ultimately determines whether people are undergoing normal or optimal or pathological ageing. A stressed-out mind affects the body and vice versa.

Optimal ageing can be achieved if we are able to break the vicious cycle of mental stress causing physical tension which in turn impacts further to mental stress and so on.

Let us examine a few points that could be contributing to your present fretfulness. There are these five components of effective interpersonal communications. If you feel you are not reaching other people, don't be quick in blaming them. Look in the mirror first and decide whether you are partly at fault.

Self-concept

The most important single factor affecting people's communication with others is their self-concept – how they see themselves and their situations. People's beliefs about themselves are determining factors in their communicative behaviour. A person's self-concept is *who* he or she is.

A strong self-concept is necessary for healthy and satisfying interaction. But this self-concept should be devoid of narcissistic delusions or fabricated spin.

Narcissists perceive themselves as perfect and are therefore arrogant. Thinking themselves special, they have unreasonable expectations of how they should be treated – a failure to meet their demands is immediately interpreted as an attack on their importance. Narcissists indulge in subtle but persistent focus on themselves, incessant self-praise, constant exaggeration of achievements and the studied pretence at being more important and more successful than they actually are.

Listening

If you have been listening to the people around you, the world would have been less trying for you. A good conversation, even when peppered with arguments, lifts the day.

Listening is a process that integrates physical, emotional and intellectual inputs in a search for meaning and understanding. Effective listening occurs when the receiver discerns and comprehends because he has used a "Third Ear". This means the listener follows not only the words but also the meaning behind the words. The "third ear" hears what is said between sentences and without words; it grasps what is being expressed soundlessly and what the speaker feels and thinks. Listening is not a passive process.

In our middle years, we will gain a lot if we talk less and listen more. Here are ways of increasing our essential listening skills:

Attend physically – Our posture conveys our willingness to listen. Sitting or standing, we shouldn't be posturing ourselves only for our comfort and convenience. We should face the other person fully and either incline the body forward (when seated) or move forward (when standing). This posture demonstrates to the other person that we are ready to hear what is about to be said.

Attend mentally – This involves the senses, especially the eyes. We communicate attentiveness when we maintain eye contact with the other person.

Suspending judgement – Temporarily suspend our own thoughts on the matter being discussed. Let the message being imparted sink in first, without trying to make decisions about it while it is being relayed.

Resist distractions – Just as you need to resist the judging voice within you, you must also resist outside distractions. Position yourself to avoid noise, other people or anything that would take you away from the person and the discussion being pursued.

Practise waiting – Wait a few seconds before responding in any way. You are likely to see a big difference in what you could say straightaway from what you will say after waiting a full 10 seconds. Check yourself out. See if those things you say right away *close off* - or *open up* - the person with whom you are talking.

Repeat the content – Repeat or re-state what you heard him/her saying and respond to physical cues. Observe the posture and energy level of the other person – are they consistent and congruent with what is being expressed?

Respond to the other person's feelings – Listen with empathy. That is, communicate respect even though you may disagree. This way, others will express themselves with less fear of ridicule or retaliation.

Clarity of expression

Many people find it difficult to say what they mean or to express what they feel. They often assume that the other person understands what they mean, even if they are careless or vague in their speech: "If it is clear to me, it should be clear to you."

We should have a coherent picture in mind of what we are trying to express.

We should be able to clarify and elaborate what we say.

We should be receptive to the feedback we get and use this to guide us in our efforts to communicate further.

Coping with angry feelings

The bottled-up anger we have been carrying through the years – caused by incidents and people we still resent to this day –

reflects our inability to deal with anger. The situation is further exacerbated because of the daily occasions for ill-feeling.

Many people suppress anger, fearing the other person will respond in kind. They tend to believe that communicating negative or unfavourable emotions will be divisive. This is not to say many people are a hundred per cent peace loving. Often, they keep their irritation to themselves and respond in a passive-aggressive manner. Take a husband who resents his wife's mindless social calendar. He could very well express his disapproval but does not. Instead, he resorts to jokes. "Did you say you wanted a book that would make you cry?" he asks a woman across the dinner table. Then he pursues: "Let me show you my chequebook. It is a definite tear-jerker."

The same man might be a total terror in the office, focusing his pent-up resentments on other people, like messengers or personal assistants. His anger may erupt at everyday events that frustrate him – a mistake by his secretary – rather than the true source, which is the wastefulness of his spouse.

How can you manage anger?

Objectively:

Anger is natural and a part of you.

Your anger is a signal about what is happening around you.

Your anger could help you know yourself better.

Your anger tells you to protect yourself.

Your anger tells you to make necessary changes or adjustments in your life.

The reasons for your anger could be shared with those who matter to you.

It is important to remember that you *choose* to be angry and to react as you do. When you allow your anger to take control of your logic and reasoning, you become powerless. You need to express your sentiments to others in a manner that could influence, affirm, re-shape and change them for the better.

You need to express your anger constructively.

Be aware of your emotions.

Admit your emotions. Don't ignore or deny them.

Accept responsibility for what you say or do.

Examine your emotions; don't seek for a means of rebuttal to win an argument.

Is there an accurate match between what you are saying and what you are experiencing.

Integrate your emotions with your intellect and your will.

Emotions should not be repressed. They should be identified, observed and integrated.

Self-disclosure

Self-disclosure is the ability to talk truthfully and fully about oneself. An individual will relate to another person only if he or she can engage in self-disclosure. This is a mutual process. The more I know about you and the more you know about me, the more effective and efficient our communication will be. We will understand only as much of ourselves as we've been willing to communicate with others.

What blocks the process is the deep-seated need to be liked, accepted and admired. As we go through life, we must learn to rid ourselves of masks.

Maturity enables us to present ourselves to others without the fear that self-disclosure will keep them from fulfilling our need to be accepted.

It is sad to note that one's chronological age does not guarantee maturity. There are 40-year-olds who act like brats; these are the middle-aged citizens who find ageing trying and taxing.

But what is maturity?

The ability to control negative emotions like anger and settle issues without violence or destruction.

It is the patience and the willingness to pass up instant gratification in favour of long-term gain.

It is perseverance, the ability to sweat out a project or a situation in spite of opposition and discouraging setbacks.

It is responding to the needs of others, sometimes at the expense of one's own desires or wishes.

It is the ability to make a decision and stand by it. The

immature spend their lives exploring endless possibilities, then, do nothing.

It means dependability, keeping one's word and coming through a crisis.

AGEING & THE MEDIA

The process of ageing starts from the day one is born. This is a patently obvious fact we often forget. "I'm growing old," a woman sighs. So is the toddler she is guiding through the park.

In the past, people talked about the world as the legacy an older generation would leave their progeny. No longer. The young have taken possession of their surroundings. The environment is awash with youth culture.

Societal factors have determined the negative view we have of getting older which, as the years go by, is being carried to ridiculous lengths. So much so that someone who is about to turn 30 could experience unwarranted anxiety!

Gerry, 34, recalls: "I suffered very bad anxiety attacks when I was 28 years old. I was in advertising and one day it occurred to me that most of the people I was working with, in and out of the industry, were only in their early or mid-20s. I was getting old! I started wondering how I would fare in my 30s. I lost all perspective. I was doing well and my superiors – who were in their 40s – couldn't understand what was happening to me.

Now, I think the advertising copy I was producing then must have got to me – products that promised eternal youth."

Media have had a role in the relentless pursuit of youth and the marginalisation of the ageing. Generally speaking, advertisements today are addressed to "people with disposable incomes" and would-be consumers aged between 21 and 45.

Insurance companies start asking more questions and require proof of reasonable health when one is past the ancient age of 50. Agents talk about "people of insurable age".

What about the beauty business? When cosmetic companies remember people beyond 50, the advertising copy invariably includes the nudge: *You don't have to look old!* Or, *70 is the new 60!* And *50 is the new 40!* On and on the self-deluding catch-phrases get spouted. A number of broadcast journalists are virtual propagandists for cosmetic surgeons. If the reconstructed, stunned face belongs to a newsreader or an opinion-maker, what subliminal message gets imparted? Shame on wrinkles, eye bags and ageing spots!

GOING BEYOND APPEARANCES

Great strides towards the improvement of societies have been made. The leaps that medical science has taken over the years have saved and prolonged lives. We have stopped saying some people are either "weird" or "loony" because we now have names and explanations for the disorders that trouble them. This has given us a deeper understanding of others and given more room for compassion. Health issues are at the forefront of many discussions and there are countless opportunities and options open to people aspiring for continuing vigour.

It is now so much easier to reach family and friends. Technological advances enable us to see people across the globe when we call them for a leisurely chat. We get instant news and we are bombarded by tons of information about so many things. We can proudly say that we are aware of a thousand and one topics.

The more important facets of ageing, however, appear to be slower in gaining society's attention. By and large, the focus has been on the physical side – cosmetic surgery and procedures, better hairstyles, aids for baldness, anti-wrinkle creams, weight loss programmes, fashion and exercise regimens that could make one look ten years younger.

Not much is said about the need to marry the physical and the mental requirements so that the ageing person could view his or her reality from the same vantage point. The 70-year-old person who wishes to be truly at peace with the world while at the same time spending a fortune to look 50 is missing the point. How can you say you are really content if you cannot accept the basic fact that 70-year-olds have multiple wrinkles?

You have to be on the same page as your current reality.

People react differently to ageing. Some people shy away from thoughts of old age – their own – for as long as they can. Eventually, reality catches up with them and they spend the last years only ruminating about the years when they were physically and mentally stronger and more independent.

There are those who look at ageing as a new adventure. Remember the man who said that an adventure is nothing more than a sum of inconveniences viewed rightly?

Elderly people suffer losses, either their own good health or through bereavement, but most manage to retain their sense of self. They navigate their way through life accepting that slippery slopes, together with calm, peaceful gardens are part of the territory. They see that growing old provides them the opportunity to learn more about themselves and this should be accepted graciously rather than dreaded.

The renowned French poet and novelist, Anatole France, put it most graphically. "All changes," he wrote, "even the most longed-for, have their melancholy; for what we leave behind is part of ourselves; we must die to one life before we can enter into another."

It was the melancholy Bill felt at 39 as he experienced a shift in attitude towards events in his life. "I was an only child and while my parents did not particularly indulge me, I did not have to learn the lesson of sharing," Bill volunteers. "We were a modest family and while I had a second-hand bicycle, I didn't have to wait for my turn to use it. It was the same with everything else. I didn't have an older brother who passed on old shirts to me. My bedroom was small but it was all mine. So I grew up rather possessive of my territory and I thought that as long as I did not bother other people and they didn't bother me, it was fine. I had a number of early relationships and they all failed. I didn't give much thought to them and found it easy just to move on. However, when I was 37, I became attracted to the girlfriend of a very good colleague. Fortunately for me things didn't work out between the two of them. My colleague was devastated by the break-up and I felt very sorry for him. After a year or so, I ran into his ex-girlfriend and she and I started seeing each other. I was very happy with Carolyn but it was the first time in my life when I stopped in my tracks and wondered about the quality of the happiness I felt. It was different. It was a confused happiness. I spoke to an old mentor about it. He suggested it might have something to do with the memory of my colleague's misery when he and Carolyn broke up. My mentor was dead right. I wasn't on a guilt trip, nothing like that. It was just that I finally saw, at 39, that my happiness could never be absolute because it could derive from the unhappiness of another. It was quite a shift for me. Prior to that, I thought I was an island. Things happened to me alone. I didn't give much thought to how other people felt."

The discovery that one thing leads to another, that the events in the world are often interrelated and that there are no absolutes are signs of a developing maturity.

As we age, these realisations get clarified for us through various experiences. How we absorb the lessons determine the trajectories of our later years.

I'M TOO BUSY RIGHT NOW BUT...

The "heaviness" that leaves us feeling out-of-sorts despite being physically healthy is often caused by unprocessed negative emotions. In other words . . . old justifications for all these sins of omission, anger, grudges and regrets.

We don't feel centred.

De-cluttering life takes time and effort. Resolving difficult issues and going beyond why we cannot come to terms with certain episodes in our lives call for the revisiting and the re-examination of the past.

The process, by necessity, is protracted. Reconciliation is a long-drawn course where we may have to be guided through past events, choices we'd made, roads we'd taken and transitions we'd managed. Unravelling the twisted skeins that have oppressed us in the past and are persisting to control the present may take more than weeks or months to do.

More often than not, we need the guidance and the assistance of other people to resolve certain issues.

Close relatives, trusted friends and mentors may be able to help. In certain cases, the subject may encounter extreme difficulty in sorting out confused emotions. Counselling may be required. But the decision to seek professional help is always up to the individual.

Meanwhile, as we navigate our way towards congruence and

self-awareness, there are strategies we can apply to our daily lives to make our current reality, our mid-life, a little brighter, and a little lighter.

STRATEGIES FOR THE PRESENT

Know exactly where you are now. Assess your current reality. For example: I am 39 years old. I'm an accountant in middle management. I am now divorced, after nine years of marriage. I live alone in a two-bedroom unit in the city. I have a mortgage to pay for the next six years. Based on my last medical check-up, I have a clean bill of health.

Say what you envisage for your future. I want to do some travelling in the next two years. Of course, I hope to re-marry. I'm grateful my ex-wife and I did not have children. But I would like to have a child someday.

Add to this how well (or otherwise) you are doing at present. If I'm careful with my money, I can manage pretty well. I have some very good friends. But I wish I were happier.

Future strategies will succeed only if you make a real commitment to your plans. This is not like all those half-baked resolutions you undertake on New Year's Eve, the ones that get discarded by mid-January.

Perhaps one of your problems is the inability to see things through to completion which has resulted in a number of heartaches. There may be underlying reasons for this incapacity but they are, as we've indicated earlier, to be tackled by another and more in-depth study.

Discovering your personal vision. Have a purpose for living. While it is sometimes advisable to take one day at a time especially during a crisis, you should not be shackled to a survivor's mentality of living only from day to day. Your vision is the cornerstone of your vitality and creativity. Be guided by memories of events, from childhood on, when you felt most joyful and fulfilled. Perhaps your restlessness will be eased if you start doing community service, for instance. Or your work could be keeping you away from your interest in music. You need not resign from your job but you could surely find ways of re-kindling a passion that had once given you much consolation.

Look after your financial well-being. Be truthful. How much are you worth or how much do you owe? Avoid further debts and do away with your concertina of credit cards. Don't spend money yet to be credited to your account. Remember that, ultimately, it is character that truly attracts and inspires, not fast cars, not flashy jewellery and certainly not the large house with the massive mortgage. Live within your means. Lessen your monthly financial debits and you will start feeling less irritable. If your job has taken you to another state or country, review your financial chart and make sure that whatever additional financial gains earned are not squandered buying countless mementos– exotic rugs, exquisite vases, old restored cabinets – that may not even fit the home you return to in a couple of years.

Live in the present. Often we dwell too much in the past and either worry or dream excessively about the future. Then we end up failing to appreciate the present. Our lives can be divided into three columns: the past (memories), the now (this moment) and the future (anticipation). We often miss out on the significance of the now – the moment – because we allow the ghosts of the past and the uncertainties of the future to overlap with what is currently happening.

Eating, reading a book, viewing an exhibit or watching a parade, our minds digress, comparing the present with what is past or hankering for what is absent. We are never fully settled in the now.

Working on our focus will make the present more meaningful for us. Our enjoyment of conversations will increase. We'll catch more nuances from the things we view. We'll find more delight in the food we eat. The present will be more pleasurable and there will be less room for regrets. Consider this case:

"My wife Fiona and I were together for five or six years and we had a daughter, Leanna. Somehow, I could not get over the fact that my in-laws thought – they certainly showed it – that Fiona was marrying beneath her station. When Leanna was born, the in-laws tried to make amends. I decided, however, being civil was the best they could do if they wanted to remain in contact with Fiona and their granddaughter. I could not fault my wife. She was very organised and ran a beautiful home; she was very creative. But I remember times when in the middle of a beautiful Sunday roast dinner I'd get into a sulk and become morose. This could be triggered by my mother-in-law calling up to say she was coming over the next day or Fiona mentioning an email from a cousin who was renovating a house in Toronto. I couldn't help it. Out of the blue I'd recall the snootiness of her family and decide that if we were caught in a battle of wills and she were made to choose, Fiona would leave me for them. Fiona and I often ended up arguing. She accused me of paranoia and calling her the Queen of Pretence. To her credit, my wife would speak up after such appalling incidents and say we should resolve the issue. I was younger then and stubborn. I refused. We ended up arguing again. She was bewildered and could not fathom my behaviour. Frustrated, she once said, "But am I not here? What do you want?" She stayed three more years but left because, she said, she had failed to expunge my demons. We were divorced five years ago. I still miss her. I now see I could have appreciated more the present that she was trying to shape with me instead of being resentful of her background and being fearful she might disappear in my life. I am 43 now and alone."

Learn how to receive graciously. Receiving here does not always refer to gift-wrapped presents. There are gestures of assistance, morsels of advice and compliments. There are people who will never ask for directions even if they have been driving around in circles for the most part of an hour and will get upset when somebody (who may be on the brink of nausea) suggests they should ask the assistance of the man walking out of the grocery store.

It is disheartening to hear things like:

My daughter-in-law makes her four-year-old son call us every Saturday without fail. It's her way of ingratiating herself. She's manipulative.

Isn't that statement infuriating? A four-year-old child calls – why can't the gesture be accepted with some magnanimity? Just concentrate on your grandson's voice and be happy you have an innocent child greeting you on a Saturday morning. Think of the other side of the coin. You could have ended up with a proud daughter-in-law who would prevent you from hearing from your son and your grandson. Count your blessings.

I wish they'd stop giving us presents. We feel under an obligation to give something back.

If people want to give you presents, be grateful they think you are worthy. You are under no obligation to repay them. If your reading is right and the gift giving stops because you didn't bother to give something back, it's still no skin off your nose. But telling well-meaning people to stop remembering you is hurtful.

I wonder why they want to drop by out of the blue. Purely a social call, they say. I bet it's an overture. Watch out; they might be asking for a loan.

Do you like these people? If you don't, you can always excuse yourself and say you cannot see them. Why have you attached a negative meaning to the proposed visit? Are you perhaps the type who remembers people only when you need something?

You think those curtains are beautiful? We got them from a bargain basement!

The person didn't ask you how much the curtains cost or where you got them.

Most of us would rather be givers and are very awkward when it comes to being recipients. This could stem from pride (we want to have the upper hand in an association or we don't want to be indebted to anyone). Or we are simply needy people who long to be needed and therefore prefer giving endlessly.

Accepting with grace is hard for people who suspect that gifts or gestures come with an ulterior motive on the part of the giver. An unwillingness to receive something without reading into it a hidden agenda on the part of the giver suggests an ungenerous and untrusting nature. Or, it could be a sign of low self-esteem where the awkward recipient doesn't feel worthy of positive gestures from others.

Just stop saying:

You should not have bothered.
Oh I hate gifts. You embarrass me!
Now what do I give you?
This is too much!
You don't have to give me anything.

They are all ungracious statements that embarrass or hurt the giver. Learn to receive with grace and say thank you. This habit will make the present better for you because you put a stop to negative thoughts and in the process start feeling good about yourself.

Concentrate on the positive side of an experience. Often we are unable to recollect clear and coherent experiences because we view them through layers of clashing emotions. You should begin the habit of weeding out the negatives from an event that otherwise would glow with positives. For instance, once every month, you go to your father-in-law's house for Saturday lunch with the extended family. You dread this gathering because there is one brother-in-law who is – and this is your considered opinion – the biggest brag in the universe. Otherwise, everything else is fine. The food is excellent. The conversation is generally friendly and intelligent. Your children play happily with their cousins. Your wife laughs easily with her siblings.

Aren't you then cheating yourself of a pleasant time because you have narrowed your attention on someone who may not even know about your irritation? Make a conscious effort to pay more attention to the fine food, the sound of children playing and the laughter around you. Soon, you'll be able to neutralise the bragging brother-in-law and he may stop all the nonsense because he will realise you couldn't care less about his car/his promotion/ his renovated patio or his trip to Alaska.

In consciously re-adjusting your otherwise negative view of a situation, you are actually allowing yourself to enjoy the intensity of the present and are putting more value in the experience.

Occasionally do something different. You can discover something new or add spice to your surroundings if you are willing to deviate from habit or routine. For example, you can decide to do something different with your garden or add brilliance to your balcony. You don't have to live only with blue hydrangeas. Think of adding something creamy-white (Queen Anne's lace, gardenia, hibiscus, calla lily); clear yellow (sunflower, rose, gerbera) and deep-red purple (Syringa, geraniums, azaleas) to the setting.

Do you regularly drive the 20-minute distance to the supermarket? Why don't you walk one day or take the bus? You will surely notice many things you miss when you are driving.

Take a different route next time you drive to visit a friend.

When you next eat out, why consider ordering something other than fish and chips?

You don't have to go to Bali for every holiday.

Are you a late riser? Set your alarm clock for a very early morning start. Begin by discovering the colours before sunrise. Later you may study how they contrast with the brilliance of sunset.

The world – yours – is full of unexplored stuff. But access to it has been restricted by your rigorous habits and routines. Why must you see a movie every Saturday? Why not plan a picnic instead? Why are you always sending carnations to your aunt? She might be pleased to receive a pot of cymbidiums. Why don't you go out for a stroll after dinner instead of returning to Twitter? How long has it been since you saw your own handwriting? Try writing a letter. If that's too much, send a couple of postcards to friends. Surprise them.

Re-discover the riches in your surroundings. We get jaded by our environment and end up taking for granted the things that should enrich us daily.

Consider taking a pause and looking more closely at a number of things that have surrounded you for years. A picture hanging in the living room, for example. When was the last time your eyes lingered on it? Look at it now and remember why it is there.

You'd probably be reminded that it was a gift from your wife and your children when you turned 40. The warmth and the affection that enveloped that episode are abundantly returned to you and the painting regains its brilliance.

Experience goes beyond the visual. Try to look beyond appearances. The ennui that regularly visits you is likely to lift if you take your attention off yourself and your complaints and notice the people around you instead. The grocer, the tailor, the seamstress, the mailman, the librarian and your colleagues (if you are still working) – have you ever wondered about their lives beyond the exchange of perfunctory greetings? Beneath the apparent politeness, have you considered that they are carrying on as best they can despite problems that may be larger than boredom issues? This exercise would make you check back a sharp rebuke when the cashier trainee makes a mistake or the librarian seems a bit distracted. Since she'd always been alert all other times, there must be a reason why she's miles away today. You need not know why – we are not suggesting you become nosey – but you could at least be patient.

Decide to be more active. Remember what you were told as a child: go out and enjoy the sunshine. Some of us had to be cajoled into doing it but the result was always positive. If you are in good health, pursue an exercise regimen that makes you pleasantly tired.

If you've been sedentary, you have to pace yourself. Seek the advice and the suggestions of a health professional. Stop saying you are getting on. Don't wait for things to happen. Make things happen.

Don't follow the example of those who work and live for the one big dream they'd allow to hatch only after retirement. Live little dreams now.

More importantly, keep your mind active. Get interested in your environment. In your walks, pay more attention to your surroundings. Visit a plant nursery in your neighbourhood and start getting acquainted with bushes, shrubs, succulents, bracts and so on.

Time yourself when you do the crossword puzzle. When you listen to music, try to distinguish the instruments from one another. When you look at a picture, think about why you like or dislike it. Read.

Start listening. Whether you are merely exchanging notes or arguing a point, it is important that you follow the nuances of your conversations with other people. Listening with half an ear leaves you feeling both dissatisfied (with the encounter just concluded) and a bit guilty (for having been disrespectful towards the other person).

Keep your word. Don't make a promise just to get out of tricky situations. This goes for small and large issues, like taking your wife on her dream holiday or cleaning your garden shed. Don't promise the children anything if you aren't sure of meeting your obligation.

Stop using your job or your awful memory every time you break your word. If you utter a promise today, write it down. Have the grace to visit the page until you've translated the promise into reality. This is very good discipline and will make you ultimately feel better in yourself.

Set aside specific times for reflection. If you feel too rushed in the morning, do so after you return home in the evening or after all your chores are done. Review the day.

So the day didn't go your way. Don't dwell on it. Stop searching for excuses. It is done. Forgive yourself. Give your mind a rest.

Accept that it is an imperfect world and while you are expected to do your utmost best, there is no perfection. Therefore, when other people make mistakes, forgive them too. Like you, they aren't perfect. Point out the errors and then move on.

Draw up an inventory of the pluses and the minuses in your life. Consolidate the positives, like friendships and interests that still keep you engaged. Be brutal about the negatives. Include in the spring-cleaning the old, old issues that still make you uneasy and fretful, like festering issues with relatives and regrets over misdeeds that ruined relationships. Make a commitment to address them. Make time to work towards ego-integration and self-awareness.

CHAPTER 3

VITAL: SELF-AWARENESS

We have the unspoken desire to be at peace with the world. We have not totally expelled residues of past mistakes. Now and then we still wrestle with questions. Had we been fair? Had we tried our best? Could we not have been kinder? The wish for synchronicity follows us everywhere.

How can we rid our lives of angry shadows?

Where is the path to optimal ageing?

LIFE SKILLS

Every stage in life has to meet requirements for us to develop into functional, healthy human beings. Apart from food and shelter we also need nourishment for our psychological well-being.

As we grow up, our parents and guardians imbue us with ideas on the responsibility of meeting these developmental requirements. Ideally, this changeover should be as seamless as possible.

For example, an exit from the family home should cause no rancour on the part of either parents or children. It must be treated as a healthy progression – a credit for a couple's parenting role and an exciting celebration of a transition into adulthood. But if the parting is marked by intense drama – an angry father throwing out his son or a mother claiming loudly about abandonment by her daughter – a rupture occurs. This breach of peace should be resolved speedily because, if allowed to fester, both parties will feel the sting of their sores for years to come.

By adulthood in our 30s, we should have begun consolidating ideas about what's best for us going forward. For instance, we should have:

Developed and honed our communication skills;

Learned mindfulness in our dealings with other people;

Improved our money management;

Kept up re-examining our levels of expectation;

Discovered the difference between mere activity and actual achievement;

Sorted out our priorities and cultivated the grace and flexibility for compromises;

Learned to calibrate our mental and emotional health by making sure that what we think and what we feel don't clash;

Seen and experienced the joys of companionable silence.

These are life skills we need in all the succeeding chapters of our adult lives.

Communication skills. If we don't speak up and articulate our beliefs and our feelings, people will take it for granted we concur with whatever it is they are saying or doing. People are not mind readers. It is clearly not their fault, should they carry-on expounding subjects on which you strongly disapprove, when all along you have failed to indicate the areas bothering you. Don't drop hints. Don't be facetious or sarcastic. Don't use the passive-aggressive weapon of sick jokes. Don't grunt or grit your teeth or bunch your fists. Just state your case. A reasonable person listens.

All cooperative action is dependent upon effective communication. Interpersonal communication, broadly defined, refers to any verbal or non-verbal behaviour perceived by another person. It is both a *message* and a *signal* sent by an individual or a party to a receiver (or receivers) with a conscious intent of affecting the receiver's behaviour.

Effective (or successful) communication exists between two parties when the receiver interprets the sender's message in the same way the sender intended it.

Miscommunication happens in every relationship. But you can minimise its frequency and its impact on your relationships. There is a tendency for us to underestimate the other person's capacity to understand. It is a shortcoming we may have picked up as youngsters living with our parents. Did you have a mother who dented the car, rushed it to the repair yard and told you not to mention it when your father returned home from an overseas trip? Because, she said, your father would get upset; *he would not understand.* Did you have a father who took you to the pub and suggested afterwards, "Don't tell Mum I brought you here or we'll both be in trouble"? In both situations, the parents are portrayed as incapable of accepting simple facts – a dented car, a visit to the pub – without turning into monsters. In both cases the children have been co-opted to lie. Repetitions of the examples given here can result in children growing into adults believing the veneer of peace sustained by lies is preferable to the testing opportunities for real growth afforded by uneasy truths.

Of course it must be borne in mind that communication is not limited to complaints and differing opinions. We must also convey the warm and loving thoughts we have for others. We must tell people how grateful we are for what they have done for us. We must extend the best wishes and kind regards we have for friends and acquaintances.

Speaking up is just one face of the coin; the other is *listening.* Have you been at a dinner table where everyone seems to be talking at the same time? Have you ever witnessed TV panel discussions where moderator and panelists interrupt one another? The cacophony reminds one of fishmongers arguing deals in wet markets. Sometimes we end up in arguments where one says, "But I told you!" If we had been listening, we perhaps would not have been debating so heatedly. All of us need information that can be acquired only by listening.

Mindfulness is the awareness of our inner and outer selves that puts us in tune with our surroundings. It keeps us in touch with our emotions. Knowing ourselves means having set our standards, benchmarks and boundaries. These guide us when dealing with others. We nurture friendships that help us grow further and move away from negative associations.

Money management. We should be reasonably skilled at this by now.

Our levels of expectation are tied up with mindfulness. Often we get disappointed because our wish lists tend to be unrealistic and not aligned with our own worth. You may wish to be a concert pianist. But if you've barely passed the yearly piano exams, you're probably better off considering an alternative direction. You could end up being a very happy engineer who plays the piano reasonably well. This isn't a far-fetched illustration since most of us start with a number of burning ambitions. Your dream of the concert stage could very well be challenged occasionally by the vague desire to build bridges or a magnificent house on stilts. The point is, you must not think that you've failed because you've adjusted your goals. If you look more closely at situations where you opted to make adjustments, you'll find they were episodes that got you aligned with various realities in your life. Do you remember the feeling of relief afterwards? This realistic and practical view of the world makes for an easier passage to the middle years. If no ruptures occur in middle age – or, if there are and these get resolved – one can expect a more comfortable ageing. Many complications arise when we assign ourselves certain objectives that are way above our capacities, whether these be talent, skill or financial. Let's look at Dan's situation. He is a dissatisfied 35 year-old accountant because his dream Ferrari is not within his reach. So, what he does is job-hop, drink excessively on weekends and invest heavily on lottery tickets. Obsessions don't just drop from the sky. Dan's fixation with Ferraris may have resulted from an earlier trauma. Perhaps he became convinced the first great love of his life dumped him because he'd been driving his father's utility van. Whatever, Dan had not confided his troubled thoughts to an effective adviser. A range of alternative reactions would most certainly be on offer to Dan following more considered analysis. He probably should not blame his father's utility van. Could it be that he was slovenly, looked and behaved like a slob when he was driving it? And what if Dan was neat, well mannered and thoughtful and the girl really minded going to the movies in a utility van? Then somebody should have intruded into Dan's sorrow and pointed out to him that such a person was not worth the trouble. Apart from talent, skill or financial wherewithal, there are other requirements our expectations pose before they become our reality. *Discipline and commitment* are two of them. You may have the wish and the talent but do you have the discipline to follow through? How committed are you?

Critical difference between mere activity and actual achievement – When we are feeling lost or empty, we tend to fill the day with unproductive pursuits just to kill time. The bustle of activity consoles us. But where does all the movement lead us? What do we achieve after the to-ing and fro-ing, the talking in circles and the contrived rushing?

Knowing your priorities and being prepared to make necessary compromises – We should have worked out the fields we consider relevant and significant to us and the objectives towards which we would, for the most part, direct our attention. However, since life should not be a matter of just *me* (or, *me* and *me*), there will be times when compromises are needed. We should be able to weigh-up situations and have the grace to accommodate the reasonable requirements of other people.

A *constant calibration of one's mental and emotional health* is required for optimal ageing. This doesn't mean hours of introspection devoted to the analysis of yourself and your desire to be perfect. That could only lead to a form of narcissistic preoccupation bound to bore your family, friends and associates. Whatever it is that's troubling you must be communicated. Problems have to be discussed. Sorrows must be shared. You have your personal rhythm and while you may every now and then be called upon to keep in step with others, you must not allow unreasonable demands to distract you from your own goals. Don't give in to emotional blackmail. Learn to say 'no'. Don't be afraid to risk being chastised or disliked or unloved by people with their own selfish agenda. Remember that it's not possible either to love or respect a doormat. It is important that you establish how far you're willing to go in accommodating other people's demands on your time and space. Likewise, in dealing with others, you should always be vigilant about overstepping lines and overstaying your welcome. All of us must observe our boundaries. Your life must be a balance between work and play. Whatever your goals, you must never lose your sense of fun.

The joys of *companionable silence* – Silence is very much more beneficial in a world that is getting increasingly noisy and intrusive. We should be able to cultivate a respect for silence; to learn that we don't have to talk incessantly or loudly to be heard or noticed. More importantly, our associations and relationships will continue to grow and flourish if we give other people sufficient room to function and hold their views. There is always the need to voice an opinion as well as to listen. This is a given. However, as an association or relationship grows, a deeper understanding of one another is achieved. With very little said, lulls in conversations can occur without one or the other side thinking something has gone wrong. People who can be together and appreciate each other without filling silent gaps with unnecessary chatter are indeed very fortunate.

RUPTURES, CRACKS AND DEVELOPMENTAL TRAPS

The path to optimal ageing is not as smooth as we would wish. No matter how diligent we are in maintaining our life skills, the world has its ways of testing our mettle.

The requirements for healthy growth and development are set from the time we are born. Babies must be fed and cared for to survive. Toddlers are helped through their initial friendships. Schoolchildren are assisted through the early learning years. Teenagers demand both attention and freedom. The process goes on.

What turns people into nags? When do we get tedious and repetitious? Why do discussions deteriorate into yelling matches?

One factor stands out through the various stages of our development as human beings sharing a planet. It pops out every now and then in our discussions, arguments and altercations: *the need to be heard, understood, accepted and validated.*

You just don't get me.
You aren't listening at all.
Why can't you see that I'm hurting here?
That isn't the point!
That's not what I meant.
You are putting words in my mouth.
How else could I explain it?
Don't change the subject.
What more can I say?
Listen and perhaps you might finally get it!

These are just some examples. There are hundreds and hundreds to illustrate the frustration of someone wishing to be heard . . . or someone who *perceives* that he or she is habitually ignored.

There are signs when things are awry. Babies cry when they are hungry or wet or want to be cuddled. Toddlers cry, too, but there are the additional tantrums. Teenagers sulk, break curfews and slam doors. Adults engage in hurtful exchanges and leave each other.

By the time we become responsible for our wellbeing, a few ruptures may have occurred in our growing-up years. These should have been addressed and resolved, thereby enabling us to move into the next phase of our adulthood. Unresolved issues block further growth and become developmental traps that we drag along as we proceed through life. Because life goes on, we continue facing more trying circumstances that need to be cleared up. If we keep ignoring the importance of such closures, we end up with a stockpile of unsettled concerns.

Bernie recalls a very bad childhood where his father was an ogre and his mother a shrew. There were constant fights over the way things were run in the house. . . how Bernie should be disciplined and over money. He couldn't wait to leave. Bernie departed home when he was 17 after one particularly heated argument with his parents. In the first couple of years, he would drop by on weekends to see whether his absence had improved things on the home front. It had not. So Bernie stopped going for a very long while. He concentrated on working and studying. He became an engineer. Then he met his future wife.

He decided to introduce her to his parents. The meeting was a total disaster. By this time, Bernie's father was very ill but very bitter and his mother made the fiancée listen to a chronicle of her son's shortcomings. Bernie decided he would no longer have anything to do with his parents except to contribute financially to their upkeep for which he was never thanked.

Even long after his parents had died, Bernie harboured a strong resentment for the way he was raised. It made him short-tempered and impatient with others. He became very rigid in his views. He didn't wish to have children. He found it difficult to communicate with his wife. Their marriage ended in divorce after eight years.

It takes moral courage to put contentious matters to bed. It's not easy to admit to errors of judgment, failures and sins of omission. To do so, however, can provide stunning rewards.

We may not be responsible at all for causing the fissures appearing in our personal geography. There are numerous examples where those suffering directly can't be held responsible for the ruptures which affect their lives so adversely in later years. Having been given up for adoption, for instance. Being orphaned at 12 years old. A mother filing for divorce when her child was barely 10. An accident, at six years of age resulting in a withered leg. Early childhood abuse.

All those ad hoc episodes disrupted corresponding developmental needs at the time they occurred. The adopted baby could be shunted aside by the unexpected pregnancy of its adoptive mother. The orphan finds himself living with very strict relatives. The 10 year-old could be the subject of a protracted custody battle. From age 6, the child with a withered leg might be excluded from many games, or be bullied by tyrannical schoolmates; even overprotected by scared parents.

Disruptions caused by the absence of love, the sudden loss of parental support, perceptions of anger or the early sorrow of a debilitating illness can mar and retard a child's progress through accepted developmental growth. Delays, thus inflicted, have various ways of manifesting themselves and should be attended to immediately the child displays negative patterns of behaviour. An adopted child may appear indifferent towards his adoptive family. The orphan may be disruptive at school. The child of a single mother may prove too clingy. The child with the withered leg may display tendencies of undermining others while keeping the façade of being overly friendly – a passive/aggressive stance. A victim of early childhood abuse is likely to be suspicious and display strong resistance to demonstrations of warmth and affection.

If the child concerned does not get proper attention and guidance to arrest disturbing behavioural patterns, a developmental trap is set and carried through the years.

Since life is constantly changing and challenging, more ruptures occur, creating additional developmental traps. Every day presents an occasion for fissures. Issues come up like weeds between untended cracks.

The electricity bill arrives in the mail. Husband and wife start arguing about it. Tensions escalate to an explosive situation where verbal abuse erupts, or one retreats into resentful silence.

At work, an already harassed assistant receives what is perceived as a denigrating memo, but is too scared of losing his job. So he shuts up. A mother may seethe the whole day because, again, her teenage daughter has ignored her curfew the previous night.

But in so many of these situations, nothing has been said or done to resolve the issues. Too often the challenged mentally throw up their hands, concluding it's not worth all the trouble.

So the load of unresolved issues carries forward. Unhealed ruptures along with set developmental traps and delays become the root cause of unease, confused discomfort and vague, lingering sadness across the ageing years.

BUT THE SUBCONSCIOUS DOES NOT LIE

We seek acceptance and approbation. We learn clever ways of getting our way. We take to heart the admonition about not rocking the boat.

Until we are about 65, we become preoccupied pursuing personal goals and working for our families. We face huge tasks and, for the most part, the "resolution of issues" is often dismissed as subjective and self-indulgent. Sometimes when the road to resolution gets patchy and problematic, we can even be accused of being unnecessarily belligerent, causing trouble and sacrificing peace. There are instances when we are told: *But that happened a long time ago. Move on!*

The demands of society for veneer politeness, the need for approval and acceptance and the fear of rejection make us assume, despite inner turmoil, a brave front in our daily lives. We wear masks as we go up career ladders. We don them to cocktail parties, barbecues, reunions and even to simple family dinners.

Move on?

Nobody can truly move on when there's unfinished business on hand. We could push it aside, hide our resentment or regret, even intellectualise or rationalise misgivings. Still, part of us would be held hostage by failure to smash our developmental traps. We could be outwardly cheerful and pretend to the world that we are all right. But what really matters is the face we confront in the mirror at the end of the day. The sorrows we have so successfully covered in layers of material possessions, the regrets we have buried under a pile of social obligations and the shortcomings we have rationalised all remain lurking. What is more, they can eventually worm their way out of the subconscious to undermine our present reality. The result is constant chatter about inconsequential matters, an injection of a sense of urgency into trivial things and a perceived state of hostage to frenetic, meaningless activity.

The case of Matt, a Pacific War veteran, best illustrates this. As a 19 year-old assistant greengrocer from country Victoria in Australia, Matt was part of an army division dispatched to Singapore to fight for king and country in 1941. When the Pacific War erupted, Matt found himself in combat in the jungles of Malaya where he was severely wounded. Later, when the British forces capitulated to the Japanese in February 1942, Matt, along with the rest of the Commonwealth troops, was first incarcerated at Singapore's Changi jail. Subsequently he was part of a large group of war prisoners transported to Japan where they became labourers on key wharves. Some died in US bombing raids. Others survived until the defeat of Japan. Matt would refer to that time as his "lost years". He returned to Victoria as a gaunt, restless, angry 23 year-old in late 1945.

His immediate world had changed in his absence. His older sister had married and become a mother. His father had had a stroke. The greengrocer had retired. His childhood sweetheart had just got engaged – the tears she shed when she said she was sorry didn't help.

To make matters worse, nobody wanted to discuss the war. Matt was told to forget the past, get a handle on things and try to move on.

He tried. He enrolled in a trade school and later became a builder. Then he got married and had a daughter. People told

Matt he should count his blessings – he now had a beautiful family, a large, well-designed home and he had money.

Matt went along with all this talk but he didn't feel comfortable in his skin. Every now and then, he found himself seething inside; he felt impatient and irked by his surroundings. When this happened, he would go to returned servicemen's hang-outs. Over lashings of beer they would regurgitate war stories and Japanese atrocity tales. From these random reunions, Matt returned home more heated and bothered. On these occasions, he would lie awake focused on his hatred towards the Japanese enemy till the wee small hours. He would rise dejected. His anger was eating him up.

It was the war. It had disrupted an otherwise simple, quiet youth. It robbed him of four years of modest but genuine delight with people he loved. War also taught him the pain of betrayal.

Matt lived through his misery until his daughter was four years old. One morning, watching her play in the park, he was overwhelmed by sadness. There he was, a man who was depriving himself of the pleasures a father should delight in because he was so mired in irrational memories of the war. He decided it couldn't go on.

What Matt did next surprised his friends. With the blessing of his wife, Matt decided to travel to Japan. He took very little money and stayed in villages. He travelled most days on foot, pursuing conversations where possible. This was in 1954. What he wanted to do, Matt confided later, was to know whether his deep-seated hatred of the Japanese, borne of the Pacific War, was justified. He also wanted to see for himself what the war did to the Japanese.

He was away seven months, subsisting on bread and rice gruel and bathing in cold water. Before returning to Australia, he went to Hiroshima and then spent a few days in Tokyo. He recognised the horrific devastation that had taken place during his years of wartime incarceration and saw countless illustrations of Allied atrocity.

Matt returned home feeling less adversarial and definitely much lighter. He also found out that he could no longer stand the repetitive war stories in the pub. He no longer wished to participate in the orchestrated anger and the way episodes of hate got more and more embroidered in the telling. Matt was ready to move on.

The physical scars stayed with Matt throughout his life but gradually he learned to push the awful war memories to the far recesses of his mind. He began to live again.

Matt and his wife were married for 61 years. It was, said Matt shortly before he died in 2009, a marriage sustained by deep understanding of each other. He was most grateful to Eva – that was her name – for having helped him get out of the hate trap that imprisoned him during the early years of their marriage.

"I could only count my blessings," Matt told his remaining friends, "after I had rid myself of the garbage of my so-called lost years."

Matt reckoned that had he not taken the step he took in 1954, he would have gone through more than 60 years of being stunted by anger and hatred. It would have affected his marriage. It would have affected the way he worked with other people. It would have affected his parenting and he could have passed on to his children an irrational fear and rejection of other people.

Stunted psychologically by war memories he could have accumulated more issues and gone on to a miserable old age. As it was, he lived a modest but peaceful existence, surrounded by family and friends who still remember him as a lucid, kindly person who inspired understanding and compassion in others.

Matt died of natural causes, passing peacefully in his sleep. He was 87.

It takes courage to confront one's demons. The process of excising them can be troublesome. Matt found he had to come to terms with the memories of the war and the new self that had emerged from it.

He didn't have much money when he went to Japan in 1954

and had only rudimentary command of the Japanese language, learned during the war years. He also missed his family badly. But he was convinced the anger that was dragging him down daily had to be expunged. He was amply rewarded for all his trouble.

TUGS-OF-WAR HARM THE INWARD WHOLENESS

Inner harmony makes us see that ageing has its fair share of rewards. This balance is determined by how truthful we have been to ourselves.

There are times when our desires clash with the requirements of others. We are placed in a dilemma because we wish to please and be appreciated by these people. The inner conflict leaves us bothered and unsure of our preferred options.

How do we resolve these endless tugs of war?

First, we should understand the phrase "going with the flow". This is what we are told when we want to pursue our interests. "Doing our thing" is not welcomed by those who want to impose their agenda on us. People even tell us: "If you go with the flow, you'll have more fun!"

It is a much-abused catch-phrase, a cliché often thrown at us by those who want us to fall in step with them.

Two things could prevent inner conflicts, the very "tugs–of–war" that leave us feeling tired for no reason or dissatisfied with our situation:

"Going with the flow."

Keeping to our boundaries.

Going with the flow refers to a relaxed way of viewing things and has to do with personal rhythm.

Our *boundaries* refer to the benchmarks and the limits we set for ourselves when dealing with others.

Being relaxed – going with the flow – does not mean giving up what we're looking for and settling for the easy alternative. It simply means not getting obsessive about finding it *right now* – the desire for instant gratification – and slipping into an easy, calm attitude where our senses get sharpened effortlessly, thus making our search a pleasant experience. Having loosened up, we see that there's no need to be frantic, no need to settle for options we have to intellectualise and rationalise later on. When we "go with the flow", our lives follow an unconfused rhythm that is ours, undisturbed by the controlling strokes of others. It is this unconfused rhythm that enables us to function to our maximum and reap well-deserved rewards.

Going with the flow also means accepting events and everyday realities with a calm disposition. This is especially important when what happens is negative – a cancellation of arrangements, a breakdown in communication, an appliance malfunction or an illness. Raving and ranting can only add more aggravation to the problem. A cool head is better able to sift through the trying details.

Keeping to our boundaries is required to retain self-integrity. Every life needs a structure that requires discipline. Rest and relaxation, leisure, spontaneity, fun – all these matter in living a full life but we can truly benefit from their therapeutic, comforting and restorative effects only if, by and large, there is order in our environment and we are pursuing worthwhile goals.

Going with the flow and keeping to our boundaries keep us whole and centred. It improves our self-esteem. We earn the respect of others.

It is not easy. It is easier to say 'yes', be swayed and to pretend we are all right when, in fact, our half-heartedness – the "tug-of-war" raging in us – is actually diminishing us by the day.

Let us say there is a report that is due at the end of the month. Your wife makes fast mental calculations and decides that you still have 22 days to complete it. She decrees that between now and then, you could actually 1) attend two anniversary dinner parties and 2) spend a long weekend with her and the children in a cottage by the sea.

Her programme clashes with what you have decided to do. It is a difficult, crucial report that you wish to approach from a calm perspective. To this end, you have planned to take a week off, potter about the garden or read in the study while collecting your thoughts. You've imagined yourself collating your notes and writing in the evenings. You've counted on the long weekend to do a final re-write. You think the extra days left could be spent going through the report and doing a final edit.

Now, what to do?

First, weigh the situation. You confront three columns: 1) anniversary parties 2) a long weekend break and 3) working on a report that would affect your standing at work.

Clearly, column 3 would be your choice. But, before making the announcement to your spouse, you must review the recent past to see how much you've invested in family life. If there'd been three long weekends so far during the year, how many of these did you spend with your wife and children? If you say, two, then it would reflect your efforts at maintaining a balance between work and family. Chances are your wife would understand your desire to devote so much time to a report.

If the answer is, zilch, perhaps you should think again. In this case, you may wish to re-examine your choice. While you may argue that your job – here represented by a report – pays for anniversary presents and holidays, it should also buy you quality time with your family.

If you and your wife communicate, it wouldn't be difficult to explain to her why you would rather stick to your planned strategy. You'd either be pottering about the garden or reading in the study because you need to be calm and collected when arguing the points you're raising in the report. You need to write in quiet surroundings. You need extra time to review what you've written – 22 days might not be enough! You'd be able to make her understand why you wouldn't wish to be distracted by anniversary parties at this point. But she'd be pleased to hear that you could use a three-day break in a cottage by the sea.

In our private lives, as in our business dealings, all parties must get a share of the positives and have a clear view of how much compromise they are willing to accommodate.

THE PATH TO CONGRUENCE AND SELF-AWARENESS

How often have you heard any of the following?

"I often feel helpless. There was a time when I didn't care."

"Isn't the world getting crazier?"

"Nobody listens."

"Respect is an alien world to my children."

"The phone doesn't ring anymore. It used to, when people needed me."

"Isn't life disappointing?"

"I'm not interested in seeing any new thing. I just want

to see and be with my children."

"Just leave me alone."

"Oh, another day. . ."

"I wish I were dead."

They are just ten of a massive collection of negative utterances that are symptomatic of a troubled ageing. They demonstrate the absence of inner harmony and the likelihood of many unresolved issues.

There are countless instances when congruence proves elusive; too difficult to make things fit. Often we shrug things off, hoping they will eventually fall into place. But a sense of peace does not just fall from the sky. Praying for harmony to happen is not sufficient. We have to work at examining our lives – an honest taking stock exercise – and thereafter endeavour to put in place that which makes things right for us.

Everyone carries certain elements of intellectual or emotional baggage. These accumulate from countless misunderstandings with family members, various sins of omission, wounding remarks uttered in impatience or anger, ugly memories of break-ups, personal grudges and deep-seated desires to feel vindicated and wreak vengeance.

But this is our problem – while we have the time, we keep postponing facing the truths that make us listless. Sometimes, we even pretend we don't remember the hurts we have inflicted on others because to recall them is painful. So we go about our daily lives and use various excuses to avoid resolving issues. We are too busy; we are not feeling well; we just don't have the time. Of course, procrastination exacts its price. We reach middle age and are fretful beyond belief.

A truly satisfying existence results when self-coherence, the integration in the here and now, is attained. Everything is aligned – the physical, the intellectual and the emotional aspects of life correspond with each other and fit, leaving us feeling whole and centered, ready for more of life. It is this required balance, this equilibrium, this sharpened self-awareness that gives us, especially in our later years, a sense of "forever-ness". When this balance is maintained, we can look to self-continuity which refers to the feeling of integrity in retrospect over our entire lifespan. In our ageing years we would enjoy the awareness of a discernible association of past, present and even future states.

To be in accord with the world, a shift must happen within us first. The heart must reconcile itself to the truths arrived at by the intellect. No diet and no amount of vitamin supplements can ease the heaviness we feel until the lessons of the intellect and the heart are meshed. Whatever it is – the absence or the death of love, career decisions gone awry, ageing – the intellect and the heart must be together in accepting the fact. The heart takes longer to come out of denial but there comes a point when together the intellect and the heart should admit: *It is what it is.*

There are demands to meet when we seek congruence.

Honesty with ourselves is the first requirement. We must truly mean it when we declare our wish for resolutions. If we mean what we say, then we must work on the desired resolution straightaway. And we should accept that we are an integral part of the process.

There must be a conscious decision to effect change or resolve issues. This is not just whim – it is a solid, intelligent step arrived at after much deliberation.

There must be commitment. We should not be half-hearted or hesitant or apologetic about what we are trying to resolve. We should recognise the substance of the issue on hand and be focused on it.

The need for a follow-through – it's not enough that we take the first step towards resolution. We must embark on the journey to integration, leaving no stone unturned. And even after we've achieved our goal, we must remain vigilant so that we don't slide back to old mistakes.

UNDERSTANDING AGEING

Ageing involves a multi-dimensional development of the individual – the biological, social, historical and psychological aspects of life. This progression occurs in the multiple spheres of life – family, education, work and leisure. Ageing treks through actions and reactions, trains of thought and choices, along with the ever-functioning pursuit and refinement of objectives. The ultimate aim of these influences is to enhance change or achieve. All point to the ever-present reality of the march of time.

Experiences don't come neatly stacked in watertight compartments. Gains and losses, growth and decline often overlap. Success in the workplace or in career may not heal the wounds of one's turbulent marriage.

Change is the constant factor we can always count on in life.

Every year brings a summary of experiences, both welcome and unwelcome. By the time one becomes acutely aware of having "travelled far" (getting old), many transitions have taken place.

The manner by which one navigates through transitions and the choices made at such crucial points determine the quality of what remains of life's journey. One pays for poor choices and gets rewarded for having settled and worked out the good options.

THE RIGHT TIME TO SEEK SELF-AWARENESS/ CONGRUENCE

Any time is the right time to seek self-awareness. The earlier it is done is the better time. The younger we are when we work at aligning the realities of our lives, the greater our progress towards more comfortable ageing. The sooner we arrive at breakthroughs the longer the pleasure we get from the things we have done and are doing.

If we decide to become better people at, say, 45 years of age, we could, in all likelihood, enjoy at least another 35 years of living in harmony with our surroundings. But, as people like saying, better late than never. What about the 82-year-old grouch who seeks congruence? Wish him luck. He should be helped to achieve the sense of peace that would make his remaining years more peaceful and harmonious than, say, the last 70.

ROD'S SEARCH FOR INNER PEACE

When Rod was 52 years old, he was diagnosed with early-stage emphysema. He ran a thriving family-owned accounting business and was financially secure. His two daughters were in their early 20s and both had moved out. His wife was in charge of the company's accounts and was very competent.

The prognosis was not dire. However, both Rod and his wife would discuss how things should be handled in case the illness took an unexpected turn. Since she had been very capable, his wife agreed that she could take over. Having reached this decision, they worked more closely together. They also saw the value of taking more time out together.

Around this time, Rod decided he needed to talk to someone less partial than his wife. He began chatting with their pastor and their family doctor who suggested he should see a therapist.

The trouble was Rod was getting depressed and had trouble sleeping. He insisted it wasn't his illness. He had accepted this and the specialists had told him he could look to many more years as long as he looked after himself. But he confided to be hounded by "a strong sense of unfinished business".

The therapist made Rod start a journal. Having been a numbers man all his life, he found this quite trying in the beginning, but soon got the hang of it. His entries were short and to the point. More importantly, heeding the words of the therapist, Rod did not fudge the sentiments he jotted down. As the entries increased, Rod noted he was returning to issues that, when recalled, made him uneasy and anxious. They were: the past animosity between he and his father-in-law and the vivid memories of himself as a bully who had made life hell for two schoolmates.

Asked by the therapist what he wanted, Rod was quick to reply – he wanted to make amends. The two schoolboys he remembered were on scholarships and came from poor families. He had discriminated against them, pushed them out of games and other activities, made them weep and almost daily reminded them they did not belong to the elite school. Rod realised that for several years now the faces of those two boys were visiting him regularly. In his dreams they were still the 12-year-olds he had traumatised but their eyes were no longer scared. They were constantly glaring back at him.

His father-in-law was another matter. In the early years of

his marriage, Rod was always at odds with his wife's father. It seemed they couldn't agree on anything, from the way Rod looked after his young family to which newspaper one should subscribe. They couldn't be in the same room for more than an hour before they started arguing. Rod's wife gave up trying to smooth things over. Ultimately, it was her idea that husband and wife should re-locate . . . three hours away from the old man by plane.

Within a matter of months father-in-law entered a nursing home with full-blown dementia. Despite the fact his wife hadn't, at any point, taken issue over his attitude towards her father, Rod became uncomfortable with the memories. His wife had been a loyal and competent partner. Shouldn't he have tried harder with her father; at least have been more courteous? Wouldn't it have been better if he had just switched off or left the room when the old man began his nonsense?

Rod discussed both the bullying memories and the father-in-law issue with his wife. He confided that the matters were really bothering and getting the better of him. Perhaps it was his health, perhaps it was also his age, but Rod said he would set out to do something about them.

Twice a year, for the next three remaining years of his father-in-law's life, Rod drove more than 800 kilometres (one way) to visit the old man in the nursing home. He would sit by the bed or the wheelchair and talk about anything. His father-in-law thought of him as a nephew or the family doctor or the plumber and conversed with him accordingly. When he rose to leave, Rod always remembered to say he was sorry for all the sad, lost years. That was the best he could do.

He was able to track down one of the boys – Jack – whom he had bullied at school. Jack had moved to Montreal where he was a practising endocrinologist.

Their meeting was cordial and Jack confessed to being taken aback by the reason for Rod's visit.

"Perhaps," Jack said, "it would help if I say I haven't even thought about you for years. Long ago, I decided to move on from that time and to work instead on bettering my lot. Of course, if you need it, I'll say it. I forgive you and now let's drop the whole thing."

The other boy, Willard, could not be found. Former schoolmates said he became a gamekeeper in Kenya. Others said he was working a massive farm in far north Queensland. Finally, he received word that Willard had been in Kenya, all right, but had been dead for several years.

Rod decided that, like Jack, Willard had perhaps not thought of him at all for years.

In all likelihood he would have reacted with much the same sentiment as conveyed by Jack.

Rod felt it was he who now needed to move on. He and his wife became active in an anti-bullying campaign in their home state.

A SENSE OF HISTORY GIVES US
A SENSE OF WEALTH

"Connecting the dots" is when we take stock of our lives – contemplate how we arrived at the present and examine what else we might do to improve our lot.

Let us take up the exercise using a trip you've taken. Let's say you and your wife went to visit some relatives in Oregon, Seattle and Vancouver. It wasn't your choice. You had hoped to spend at least a couple of weeks of your two-month sabbatical on a golfing tour with a group of friends. But your wife reminded you that your job had been taking you away from the family for most of the year. So you go traipsing around Oregon, Seattle and Vancouver with her and the children.

You eat too much and hear little. You take a few photographs and snatch a few impressions that fade rather fast. You return home and when asked how the trip had been, you say, "OK". Truth is, you really don't know how to sum it up.

You recall snatches of conversations, a particularly good dish and somebody's vibrant garden but that's about all. The experience is recalled in fragments, bits and pieces that don't amount to a failure but can neither spell success. The dots don't connect.

Compare this to a time when you took your son fishing for the first time. You recall the things he said when you were teaching him how to attach bait to hook.

You still feel a surge of joy when you remember how enthusiastic he was when the two of you were pitching the tent. You keep the picture of the first fish he caught. Your son is now 21. He remembers having caught three trevally. You remember only two but it doesn't matter.

It was a weekend when things were aligned and the two of you were both caught up in the promise of the present. Congruence had occurred. In the memory, the dots connect.

There's no age limit to being vigilant about self-awareness. It's always imperative to look into unresolved issues.

MEMORIES

A great part of earlier life is spent chasing memories. That's why we are always taking pictures, keeping records, hoarding souvenier programmes and jotting down notes.

There is a seemingly endless desire to document experiences. We think that diaries, letters and snapshots will forever give credence to our remembrances.

Over the years we accumulate a vast amout of memorabilia.

But our memories eventually catch up with us. This is another aspect of ageing. Somehow we feel compelled to sit back and sort out what has transpired thus far.

Unfortunately, most of the things we recall are vague impressions of past events that, for convenience, we categorise either as pleasant or unpleasant. But we are seldom truly touched by them.

The souvenirs are often associated with fragmentary remembrances; indeed, there are instances when we fail to remember where we got them or who gave them to us in the first place.

But if the experiences are similar to the father and son fishing episode, the person connecting the dots will be left buoyed by the fact that life, thus far, has been meaningful; the past years have been good value.

Here we should recall what we said about knowing the difference between mere activity and actual achievement. We may cram our lives with lengthy to-do lists to which only negligible emotional value is attached.

How, then, could we ever hope to remember them sharply? It is the quality of what we are left when frenetic lists get exhausted that determines the rating of our memory banks.

There's no age limit to being vigilant about self-awareness. It's always imperative to look into unresolved issues.

As we age, we see increased need for more pleasant experiences. We also acknowledge that, as in all our past experiences, good or bad, we had a part to play and therefore must recognise our share of either glory or blame.

CHAPTER 4

MANAGING ALONE

It has often been quoted: He travels fastest who travels alone. It has also been asked: But wouldn't the journey be lonely? One could argue that every journey has its fair share of loneliness and that travelling could be lonelier when one is on the road with the wrong companion.

–Bill, 53:

"My friends say I'd be better off married. I'm thankful that since we're all getting on, they are running out of blind dates for me. I don't think marriage was ever on the cards for me; otherwise it would have happened years ago. I've found it difficult to connect – I've always been set in my ways and now that I'm 53, I would find it doubly hard to accommodate somebody else's oddities. All my past girlfriends complained about my attitude of – it's my way or the highway. My longest relationship was with a very caring woman who never questioned my imperiousness. I had very deep affection for her but found that I preferred it when we had company. Otherwise, it was very dull. I live simply and like my schedule. I get impatient with trivialities and marriage, as

I see it, is littered with them. I have a good job and with the inheritance from my parents I could live to my 80s without having to struggle. I like returning home to find the things I'd left are still where I expect them to be. Nobody reorganises my life in my absence. No neatness freak sorts out the chaos only to tell me at the dinner table what a scatter bug I am."

–Barbara. 62:

"After 38 years of marriage, my husband died, quite suddenly, from a massive heart attack three years ago. Although marriage was contentious for the most part, I find myself still mourning his passing. Our four children are grown and it's a consolation for me that my only son and his family live two blocks away. Last year I sold the big house and moved to a much smaller townhouse. My husband had looked after the finances throughout our married life and the thought that I might run out of money spooks me. I'm a chemist and still have three years of working life ahead of me. I don't think I'd ever live with any of my children. My husband was a control freak and I'm just beginning to appreciate the quiet that greets me when I push open the door to the bedroom. There's no one carping or hectoring. I loved my husband but I also love the thought that I'm beginning to get out of his shadow."

–Nick, 48:

"When I was served the divorce papers, I was totally devastated. The fact that it was I who had walked out months earlier didn't matter. I didn't contest anything. We'd been fighting for years. I wanted to keep the acrimony contained. She got the house and I

gave her full custody of the three boys. I was no saint. I was what women like calling a very good provider. My ex-wife could not fault me when it came to providing. But over the years I'd had three affairs and I guess I was pretty careless. She accused me of humiliating her. After the third fling, she just developed into a neurotic monster who thought I would bed every single woman I talked to for more than five minutes. She became insanely jealous and life became intolerable. I looked for ways to escape from her outbursts but I ran out of places that were acceptable to her. I used to get dead drunk with her own dad in the guy's own den. That's how bad it was. It was her jealousy that drove me away. I'm seeing somebody now but I don't think I'd ever live with anyone again."

–Lillian, 36:

"I have just crawled out of a four-year abusive relationship. Dean never physically hurt me but he was so sharp-tongued it took me weeks to recover from a verbal laceration. He had fuses and They were all short. Anything could set him off and his temper was frightening. In the beginning he would berate me in private. As our relationship grew, he became indiscreet and would just yell at me and tell me to shut up in front of other people. It's not that he supported me financially. I have my own career and earn good money. I contributed to the upkeep of our beautiful pad. The last straw was when he woke me up at 6 o'clock on a Sunday morning. He was in such a state because I had thrown out by mistake a tiny bit of cheddar cheese he had wrapped in foil the previous night. He looked and sounded horrid. But at Sunday dinner you couldn't have guessed that the man carving the roast had caused

so much emotional havoc a few hours earlier. I made up my mind that I'd been living with someone certifiable. I went to work on the Monday morning and never went back. Dean still insists he can't understand what I did."

CHANGING PERSPECTIVES

Of the major changes to have swept the world in the last half-century, nothing would be as dramatic as the shift in people's attitude towards marriage and family. Several lifetimes ago, we chose once and we chose forever. All that's gone up in smoke. We don't have to suffer lying all our lives in beds we've made. We are no longer expected to stay cocooned in a union if it oppresses us. In fact it's now our duty to sever ties that keep us from growing and accomplishing our goals.

Marriage is just one of the options open to us. Couples postpone having children, if not deciding against having them altogether. Double incomes don't necessarily get addressed to the rearing of an offspring or restricted to the maintenance of the family home. Many would rather now invest disposable incomes to personal enriching pursuits like travel and hobby farms. A wedded existence is not viewed anymore as better off and more settled than a life spent independently on one's own. People still like relationships, yes, but that's different from saying they're willing to exchange the pleasures of being single and singular to a lifetime of duty, accommodation and compromise. They call their choice "enlightened selfishness".

There are still traditionalists who insist this is a passing fad, a phase that society will eventually outgrow. That could be wishful thinking.

Urban planning and cityscapes take into consideration the requirements of single occupants. Studios, one or two-bedroom units, balcony gardens and shared entertaining areas have been meticulously designed for those who prefer the vibrancy of city life to the comforts of leafy suburbs. Futon mattresses and sofa beds are very popular. In department stores large collections of cutlery, crockery, glassware, quilts and bedcovers are addressed to the more adventurous tastes of those who'd rather be home alone.

Single blessedness is what it is often called and those who embrace it are only too happy to enumerate the pluses they enjoy. They don't claim it to be the perfect life but they celebrate the freedom to be themselves without being constantly judged or bullied into unwanted situations.

- You mull and make your own decisions. You either run away or get dragged down by them. Nobody asks, "How about me or how about us?"

- You earn, spend and save your money. You can be a spendthrift or behave miserly. You can sign small regular cheques in aid of a spastic children's school without someone suggesting the money is better off donated to the RSPCA.

- You nurture your own friendships. Nobody gets possessive and territorial to the point that you drop certain associations for the sake of keeping peace. You attend parties, go home and retire to bed without a partner yakking about how dreadful the evening has been and what awful people your friends are.

- You pursue your interests without being distracted or swayed by the preoccupations of another. You are able to dedicate your time to pursuits that are genuinely yours and don't feel torn between choices which happens when you feel obligated to be supportive and loyal. You are able to follow your own path towards personal and professional growth.

- You did not choose your family. There are always issues within a family. It's always easier to resolve them on your own, with the minimum of emotional fuss, without someone else driving in a larger wedge.

- An independent existence gives you a stronger sense of identity. You don't live in somebody else's shadow. You aren't anybody's echo. You either thrive or wilt: the choice is yours.

- You don't get embroiled in a blame game when something goes wrong. The risks you take are your responsibility alone. You're spared lines like, "I knew it wouldn't work; you should have listened to me!" Negative feedback makes a failure heavier to bear.

- You're ready to take on more risks and adventures when there's no one to hold you back with their manipulative vested interests.

- Outside office hours, you are the master of your schedule. You don't have to be back at the nest by a certain time. Nobody gives you the cold treatment if, on a whim, you ate out without phoning home.

- If you work from home, you can stay in your dressing gown the whole day without being told you are slovenly. You can eat anywhere and leave crumbs in your unmade bed.

- The TV remote control is yours and yours alone. Nobody walks into the room every now and then to ask, "Why do you like watching unmitigated misery?" Or, "What do you find so absorbing in tennis?"

- You enjoy the music of your choice and play it endlessly, without someone accusing you of lunacy.

THE FLIP SIDE

In your joy at being "your own person", you may forget the price of freedom. Being a solo dweller doesn't exempt you from a list of reminders.

- Be sure you monitor your health. The pleasures of lone, independent living are tremendous for as long as you remain healthy. Get medical insurance. Have a back-up plan in place in case you become seriously ill. Discuss this plan with your appointed support group.

- Your enjoyment gets curtailed if your finances are in a mess. Seek advice before expenses and debt overtake you. Don't keep a concertina of credit cards. Consolidate your obligations and save on interest rates. You may be alone but you are not exempt from thinking of the future.

- Who shares your deepest sorrows? When things aren't working out for you, when nothing seems to register, whom do you talk to at 3 o'clock on a cold morning? See to it that you have a back-up plan. It could be a notebook by your bed. Sit up and write down your thoughts. Don't just toss about and get sadder and angrier by the hour.

- All the independence and freedom could make you even more rigid as you age, making the world appear awry and other people, by and large, unacceptable to you. This narrows your social circle and in certain cases even results in social isolation.

- Having had your way for the longest time, you may end up with a disproportionate sense of entitlement – an ageing person who thinks, "There's only one way and it's mine."

- How do you achieve congruence and self-awareness if you don't have someone who's unafraid to point out your foibles?

- A life shared is often a life examined. There's no escaping this. The significant other appoints him/herself your conscience. But what if there's no one? You could end up with a huge pile of unresolved issues – not a good way to confront the challenges of ageing.

- How neighbourly are you? Because you are alone doesn't mean you have the right to hold all night parties, play blaring music or use your vacuum cleaner at 7 o'clock on a Sunday morning, informing the tenants in the flat below that you're wide awake.

- The fact that nobody else is around to accuse you of being slovenly doesn't give you the licence to be habitually unkempt, careless and smelly.

- A life alone can be very rewarding. But the meaningful rewards – solo risks that flourish, good friendships that get pursued without reservations, a quiet peaceful abode to return to – are the result of a self-imposed discipline.

GRIEF & BEREAVEMENT ARE FACTORS

There are times when aloneness is imposed on a person. A spouse walks out on the marriage or is transferred to a nursing home or dies. Here, a mourning period needs to be observed before one can move on and see the consolations of being single again.

No matter how poor the quality of the union has been – co-dependent, contentious, abusive, a one-way street, dull as dishwater – grief takes over when it is brought to a close.

Therese, 73, confides: "Peter went for elective surgery for moles he wanted removed but the operation was botched. I trace the deterioration of his health from that time. He started having mood swings, getting forgetful and depressed. Then it was a gradual slide to dementia. He was only 67. I was still working and watched our retirement plans go up in smoke. I took early retirement to look after him. I tried to keep him at home for as long as I could manage. Peter loved our home and would not hear of selling it. Fortunately our children were very supportive. On weekends they took turns coming over with their families to give me some time off. My daughter convinced me to hire a cleaner who came twice a week. That was a big help. We had to move Peter to a facility centre when he was 77. He was there nearly three years and died shortly before he turned 80. This was two years ago. Peter had full-blown dementia at 74 but the family home became the core of his long-term memory. I suppose it wouldn't have mattered had I sold it then right under his nose. But I couldn't do it, despite his forgetting he was part of my decision-making. That was how it was with us. It was two years after his death that I finally sold the house. I still miss him but I'm glad I did my best in looking after him."

The sense of loss we feel when a relationship ends has many layers. These have to be peeled away before we can come to terms with the new reality. We just can't hope that the pain will go away one fine day. Things do pass and time does heal but we have a major part to play before healing can begin.

When a person leaves or dies, what do we really mourn?

- **The fact that our world is changed forever.** If it's death, we mourn a permanent absence. If it's separation or divorce, we grieve the failure of a partnership on which we'd pinned so much hope. We are distressed over the fact that love could turn so disloyal or so angry or so nasty or so vindictive. The more acrimonious the parting of ways, the longer the grieving or mourning period tends to be.

People remark on how the newly widowed or newly divorced often look so good at wakes or at divorce courts.

No matter how prepared we are for somebody's departure, the exit still has an emotional and psychological impact we wouldn't have imagined. However, a survival mechanism is triggered in us at such times. It enables us to function almost mechanically – we are aware there's pain but become temporarily detached from it. The mind gets focused on other things. We notice a stain on the ceiling, the print of someone's shirt, or feel the need to make lemonade – distractions that block a full-blown, frenzied, emotional outburst. So we are able to choose a suitable tie or even laugh or apply lipstick.

Tommy was 41 when his wife died in a motor accident. He recalls: "I remember receiving the telephone call. I sat down on the edge of the bed and thought – she's dead, she's dead. But they were just words. Then I thought I wanted a cup of coffee. I made one but left it on the kitchen table. I looked out the window and decided the lawn was looking messy. I'd mown half of it when my brothers-in-law arrived. I was on auto-pilot for days."

- **The denial of a future with the person who left us, regardless of flaws in the relationship.** For a long while we may think that somewhere along the line we could have worked out the kinks. Why didn't we? We feel short-changed – it's unfair! This thought may be tinged with anger. Anne's husband announced that he wanted a divorce after 12 years of marriage. She was 37. "I could not help thinking that had we discussed things more often we could have each tried to resolve the issues troubling him. It would appear he suffered in silence. At crunch time he claimed I was too ambitious and always placed our family second to my career. I wouldn't deny being ambitious but I also cared deeply about him and our daughter. I was very upset. I was very angry. I accused him of fabricating excuses so he could be free to marry his girlfriend."

- **Regret over sins of omission.** We are haunted by thoughts that we could have done better for the other person, that we could have been less self-absorbed and less selfish. We will always feel we'd fallen short of our best. We will consider the steps that we should have taken to make the patient more comfortable, less scared and more loved. The sick and the dying only know what they expect and want – looking after them is a monumental duty that could fray our nerves. We will regret the times when we made our impatience obvious. We will rue the instances when we escaped the rigours of care giving.

Rod's wife died when she was only 34. Rod was 41. It took him many years to get over the guilt that he did not take compassionate leave in the final weeks of her life. He was vice-president of a big engineering firm. "I could have done it but I needed something to get my mind off her illness. As it was, they had to telephone to inform me her pulse had turned very faint. I rushed to the hospital to find they were trying to resuscitate her. Then she was gone. For a long time I couldn't forgive myself. I thought I had been remiss and had been cowardly."

- **Regret over things we should have said and settled.** Because we are often in denial that things are at an end, we postpone tying loose ends and giving voice to sentiments that signify our acceptance of the inevitable. Usually, the event overtakes our intention of expressing love, thanking the loved one, sharing regrets and asking forgiveness for whatever hurts we may have inflicted in the past.

Dinah, 66, is still grieving the death of her husband of 41 years. Dan died three years ago. "I guess we didn't know how to handle it," Dinah admits. "Dan and I usually intellectualised the events in our marriage. Even when he was taken grievously ill, I couldn't make myself express the sorrow I felt at the thought that he would leave us. I didn't want to sound too dramatic or maudlin. After we'd buried

117

him, I was at a loss as to how I could make up for my failure. I'd longed to tell him that I was sorry for the hurtful things I'd said during a tricky episode in our younger days when we thought we would leave each other. I wanted to say I forgive him the flaws I'd pointed out to him; I'd longed to say that, despite those, he was a good man and I couldn't have imagined a life with another. He was a good husband and a good father; he tried his best. Hearing that would have made him happy. But my arrogance stopped me from being honest with the man I'd lived with for 41 years."

- **The failure to resolve the festering issue that was the root cause of constant bickering.** In contentious relationships, we often zero in on issues that are peripheral to the very source of our major resentments. If a person suddenly makes an exit and we don't get the chance to air these grievances, we have to tackle the issues in his/her absence on our own. This takes time. For instance, somebody who has always been perceived to be in his/her partner's shadow could spend half a lifetime carping about bad temper and thoughtlessness when the actual issue is a desire to break away from oppressive control. When a complex partnership gets dissolved, the one left behind feels terribly cheated.

Karina, 58, was widowed five years ago. Her husband, Mel, had a very successful architectural practice. They had two sons. Karina asserts that her husband's mercurial temper and unreasonably high standards alienated the boys from them very early in the piece. Her regret was that she always took her husband's side in arguments, justified his outbursts to their sons and, by and large, left her children to fend for themselves against their father's rants. The sons made it known that they'd sometimes expected Karina to be on their side. When they were grown, they told her point blank about their disappointment. It became a black mark against her husband. They argued about it but the issue remained unresolved. Once widowed, it occurred to Karina that she had been unfair to both her husband and her sons. She hadn't had the guts to protest strongly against Mel's unhealthy sense of entitlement. She likewise failed as a mother who should have given her sons a fairer and more equal picture of marriage. Karina went for counselling and for more than four years she experienced riding an emotional pendulum.

"It's taking me a long time to accept that I can't undo the past. For a while I found excuses why I responded to tricky family episodes the way I did. It was only after I'd been confronted by many questions that I gradually accepted I'd been trying to protect the image other people had of my marriage. My husband and I were both successful. I'd wanted to remain part of a golden couple.

"After my husband died, my children and I suffered emotionally and psychologically. Finally we submitted ourselves to family counselling. In a number of tearful confrontations I apologised to my sons. One of them said I loved their father to a fault but they'd expected a bit of moral support from me, especially when they were teenagers. It devastated me to think that I'd been a weak wife and a weak mother.

"My sons said we should just accept the past, forgive ourselves and move on. I was very slow in taking that up. I felt very sorry for their father and I wanted to be re-assured they loved him too. My older son said, 'Mum, we love each other the best way we can. We believe Dad loved us in his own way and we'd long accepted the way he was. We loved him the best way we could and we think he knew it. But he's dead, Mum, he's dead, and you should start thinking of what's best for you.'

"There were sessions when my sons appeared very upset with me but the counsellor encouraged them to say what was on their minds. Otherwise, he said, nobody would ever get healed. My younger son said I should let go of the veneer of perfection I'd tried to put up while their father was alive. That pronouncement shook me. He said we may have had happy times but my marriage to their father was far from perfect and it was time we all stopped pretending. It was difficult to hear. It's always difficult to hear the truth.

"My children have displayed extraordinary resilience. We are closer now, as close as possible in the circumstances. I'm getting there."

BEREAVEMENT HURDLES

It is the lack of closure that makes bereavement a protracted journey back to wholeness and, hopefully, wisdom.

It is very easy to suggest mourners should move on, but there are hurdles.

- The bereaved may claim to be sad but in reality be evading intense pain by being ultra social and filling gaps with endless, determined activity. Grief gets frozen but as it hardens it blocks the path to post-bereavement growth. The mourning gets protracted.

- The bereaved may deny the severity of the unresolved issues that had adversely impacted on their lives.

- The bereaved may be fearful of what they might have to accept about themselves.

- The bereaved may be unwilling to let go of the illusions they had of the past and the lamented.

- The bereaved may feel that examining their sorrow would be disloyal to the departed.

But the immensity of grief has its way of sneaking up on us. Sooner or later we have to confront it.

We may not like the realities that can pop out while the various issues are being processed, but there's no other way if we truly wish to lay our loss to rest.

RESUMING LIFE

- There must be a conscious decision to work towards the acceptance of the new reality. If you got divorced or you've been widowed, you can't be burying the sadness in a mountain of activities and hoping you'll eventually emerge healed and all right. Turning reclusive doesn't help either. You have to get out there and learn to function on your own.

- Self-awareness is essential when you're in the midst of processing grief. You need to reflect on why you're doing what – why you are working doubly hard, why you are travelling so much, why you are throwing so many parties, why your shopping sprees are endless. More often than not, the answer is: you are evading the full-on confrontation with grief.

- The sooner you accept this fact, the better. Running away from grief doesn't solve anything. Ultimately it catches up with you and you'll find that you're not just sorrowful but bone-tired and mentally exhausted as well.

- Beginning again and doing it only by yourself is arduous business. A divorced person can't keep all the friendships established and maintained during the marriage. Widows and widowers have to learn living solo in a social set-up made up of couples.

- Sooner or later, your remaining friends will try to pair you off with somebody. This will be one of the more predictable turns in your new reality.

- It's advisable to go back slowly to activities you've always enjoyed. Keep this on balance. Feeling isolated, you'd feel most vulnerable and might get trapped in 'sorry' relationships.

- Pace yourself. Now that you have full control of your life and schedule, sit down and decide which interests you wish to pursue. You don't have to cycle or jog or play tennis to make somebody else happy with you. Make a list of what is pleasurable for you. Then prioritise your activities.

- Never be frenetic. While you're still feeling fragile, don't jump into new commitments. Grief makes us brittle and vulnerable. Our desire to get over a loss as fast as is humanly possible often leads us to settling for new arrangements without giving these much thought and thorough examination. We end up with additional disappointments. This happened to Sandra after her divorce from Jason. She says: "I was very lonely and hankered for affection. My self-esteem was battered by the heated exchanges that preceded the final separation. I wanted to prove to Jason that I could have another relationship and succeed with it. So I dated indiscriminately. I had a couple of 'sorry' relationships before I went for counselling."

- Pets help in the healing process. The fact that you have to look after them – feed them and walk them, for instance – should get you out of wallowing in dark thoughts.

- Count on your support group. By this time you should know who listens and suspends judgement. These are the people you need while you're processing your grief.

THE PROCESS

Sorrow has its way of burrowing into our bones and, no matter how strong our denials, there comes a point when we have to reach out and ask to be assisted in chipping away the crippling pain.

Clearly you can't do it alone. You will need the support and guidance of other people while you navigate your way through a highly individualised trauma. No widower could ever say, "I know how he feels." He doesn't; he wouldn't. Bereavement is highly personal and its depth and intensity are determined by the quality of the relationship and the circumstances leading up to the final loss.

There are no hard and fast rules when it comes to bereavement. Your response to it is yours alone. You may not wish to talk about how lost you feel. You may talk excessively about your story. Neither tack is preferable nor better than the other. But for your own sense of self and peace of mind, you have to work at coming to terms with the loss sooner or later. The decision when to do it is yours.

You can't put a time-frame on your healing and compare your situation to others. If Grace was able to "get over" her husband's death in less than a year, don't assign yourself a similar timetable. This is about healing, not a sprint competition. You are not Grace. The issues she had to resolve are in all likelihood vastly different from yours.

The daily trek towards post-bereavement calm is best achieved if the mourner manages to strike a balance between recognising the pervasive gloom of loss and the undeniable requirement to go on living. It is a matter of focus, a matter of deliberately assigning a time to indulge the loss and periods of intensely concentrating on life – working, cooking, looking after the dog, going out to dinner. It is difficult in the beginning but the discipline has helped a great number of people especially during the early stages of bereavement.

"It helped me in the early months after my husband passed away," says Sophie, 63. "I did not rush out in the early morning when I felt down. I would cry and cry for the most part of an hour. But crying does tire you and then I'd remember a meeting I had to attend at ten. There was no choice. I had to express my loss but I also had to get on with my life."

Honesty is a requirement in the path to post-bereavement growth. You should stop rationalising hurts and failures and evading responsibility. In Karina's case, for instance, the counsellor perceived her half-heartedness in accepting the realities of her marriage that had adversely affected the growing years of her sons. She might have been puzzled when the counsellor did not stop her children from voicing their belligerent sentiments. But how else would the three of them heal if, even from the grave, the highly successful architect were allowed to have his hold on Karina?

Karina herself had to admit her desire to remain part of a golden couple was largely an illusion. Her son suggested they should all stop pretending. Only when Karina was shaken into honesty did they score a breakthrough in the counselling sessions.

When the unresolved issues are of a magnitude such as in Karina's case, professional counselling is advised. Relatives and friends can only be a support group. They are people one can lean on. But sisters, brothers and best friends are not necessarily well placed for what is then so often required – therapeutic approaches and reality-based therapies. These work at bringing the client finally to face up to things. Extensive research in this field strongly reinforces the view that immediate family members are both ill-equipped and poorly placed for guiding a severely demoralised, tearful and resistant close relative back to reason.

Healing cannot be rushed. One day you may feel perfectly fine and the next horribly down. This is part of the process. A seesaw of perceptions occurs when you stop running about, masking your sorrow with frenzied activities. It is a sign that you've given a window to reflection, an essential factor when you're sorting out the issues that prevent you from feeling at peace with loss.

It is very important for you to keep a close watch on your health when you're grieving. While you may not have the appetite for big meals, make sure you consume food rich in nutrients. You may feel sluggish but, please, will yourself to get up and take long walks.

In an effort to avoid sad thoughts, don't tire yourself unnecessarily. If you feel too exhausted, sleep won't come easily. Gradually, as the various unresolved issues get examined and settled, you will find an instinctive need to re-organise your ideas and attitudes.

You will have to.

You cannot, by yourself, face difficult and trying situations in future with the same mind-set that was heavily shaded by the thoughts of a departed spouse.

Part of your mental, emotional and psychological de-cluttering is the task needed to relocate the departed in your personal emotional sphere. You need to put into a context the realities of illness and death. It is important you understand how and why they've left you devastated. When this relocation is done you will be able to transition and adapt to a hugely revised routine without feeling guilty or disloyal.

Around this time, you may start feeling a genuine interest in participating in life again. This is very different from the patchwork quality of those days when you sought to fill your waking hours with appointments to get out of the house and forget.

Take baby steps. Every recovery from bereavement is fragile. Slowly get used to your newly restructured life. Don't expect sadness to lift forever. You will still be occasionally lonely, as all of us get lonely. But you will have integrated the gloom and the grief of your loss so that when you sit back and remember, you aren't overwhelmed by your memories. This is the best sign that you've emerged from that long tunnel of bereavement.

GOING SOLO

One fine day, you may be surprised to hear yourself celebrating the fact that you have full control of everything – budgeting, bank accounts, whom to invite on Christmas Eve, travel destinations, where to live and the TV remote control unit. When that happens, one hopes you will also pay attention to the flip side of freedom and the reminders that should sustain its fun. Mind your finances. Be a good friend. Listen. Think of the future. Consider the environment. Turn down that blaring music – you may be alone in your home but you are still part of a teeming humanity. Respect your neighbours. Keep watch on your boundaries and sense of entitlement.

CHAPTER 5

AGEING TOGETHER

It is testing enough to face the advancing years, but the job truly gets challenging when you are committed to see the race through with someone you love. The poet Robert Browning said: "Grow old along with me, the best is yet to be." He might have added: "Meanwhile, the two of us will have to work very hard at it!"

So, how does one do this?

Men and women differ in the way they tackle ageing. Despite celebrated advances in the area of equal opportunities, there remain residues of deep-seated expectations in the minds of all genders.

A great number of men are still saddled with the idea that they have been placed on this planet to protect, procreate and provide. Over the years men may have learned to bake bread, serve a mean lamb stew and change baby diapers. In reality, many consider these merely added pluses to what they feel certain they do better – earn the bread, buy the lamb and pay for the diapers.

Homemaking is a job most men view as temporary when it is foisted on them – a two or three-year stint while the wife is doing her doctorate, or while waiting for a business venture to start rolling, or while they are recovering from a massively demanding job that was driving them to distraction. The truth is, few men are truly comfortable with the idea of being "kept" or "maintained". They would be far happier in a two-income family where the male is the better-paid party.

Women are not any better at handling deep-seated prejudices. A high achiever delivers long speeches extolling her househusband's culinary expertise, his imaginative way with the children and what a grand moral support he is to her career. Why does she have to justify the situation? She does not owe the world an explanation. But she feels she has to say she's comfortable with it; she has to worry about her man's self-esteem. Because, despite the *summa cum laudes*, the master's degrees, the promotions and bonuses, women are still viewed as worthy to be cared and provided for and protected. For why else do people say, "She has this wonderful career and a supportive husband who also provides her with everything! What luck!" Or, "She really does not have to work so hard. Her husband can keep her in the style any woman would envy." Or. "She can write those novels because she is married to a very good provider."

Society is still dragging its feet in fully accepting reversal of roles on the home front. Househusbands comfortable in their skins are still the exceptions; but even they are known to sulk or throw temper tantrums when they feel "too ignored" or "too neglected". A high achieving woman who settles for "less" is subject to relentless scrutiny. How many times have we heard this asked of a female bank executive who ends up living with her former car mechanic: "Couldn't she have done better than *that*?"

Men struggling up the career ladder or ensconced at the top of their professions don't lose sleep when they spend weekends away from home. They are irked when their wives complain about their being away too much. "Too bad," they crow, "but it's the job."

Busy women only feel guilty. "I don't think I'll be able to make the next trip," they say apologetically to colleagues. "I've been away too long." Or, "I have to be with Bill and the children."

This attitude gap, stretched by ages of societal conditioning, extends through the later years. Old men talk about being the shadow of their former selves. It takes them longer to reconcile themselves to "diminished" importance. They may travel, go fishing or play golf but all these are mere distractions. For didn't they design houses or fly planes or skipper a sloop around Cape Horn? How can helping one's wife re-pot orchids compare with the challenge of developing a position paper on *Relearning Halstedian Principles of Gentle Tissue Handling, Anatomic Dissection and Blood Loss Minimization in Operations?*

Women can be distracted from the deeper issues of ageing by flashy advertisements selling the idea that they can postpone the tell-tale signs of advancing years. They invest in anti-wrinkle creams, sign up for weight loss programmes, do Pilates, attend short courses on horticulture or French cooking or Mandarin and undertake voluntary work in hospitals, churches and galleries.

Unlike men, women find it easier to settle in less demanding schedules. They find time to glory in the comfortable homes they have helped purchase, in the victories of the children they have raised and even re-discovery of friends lost in the years when they were busy and successful. It is also part of their make-up to appreciate the perception of a back-up – a loving and capable person who is ready to save them from collapse and destruction. It is also part of their nature to be consoled by demonstrations of affection. An old woman surrounded by happy grandchildren is often happier than her old husband who is still wandering through the recesses of memory, looking for the valiant youth he once was and the great loves he had betrayed.

THE EGO

The importance of success is inculcated in us from a very young age. By the time we are teenagers, we are plagued by thoughts of what careers we should pursue in order to do justice to the dreams and expectations of our parents or guardians.

In our mid to late 30s most of us lose the inclination to look for fun in the things we do. By this time fun is equated with the frittering away of time better spent scaling social and professional ladders. Never mind our personal interests. Our discontent and aversion to business matters, we are assured, will be temporary. There are many dissatisfied lawyers about and their discontent may not always be due to daily demonstrations of miscarriages of justice. Rather it could be linked to the fact they had wanted to be actors or painters or builders but had succumbed to becoming barristers like their fathers and grandfathers. This surrender extends even to play. While, for example, we may prefer playing football or sailing with our contemporaries, our new job in real estate could see us taking golf or even lawn bowling lessons.

By the time we hit our 40s, the sell-out is complete and we are heady with thoughts of our bright futures. We now identify ourselves with desks, salary increments and company testimonials. We think of the cars we *should* drive, the wines we *must* imbibe and the trips we *have to* take. When we look back on our young lives, we talk about the times when we shone – as outstanding young rowers or as promising mathematicians or as the students most likely to succeed.

Life becomes very competitive but we find the twists and turns very engaging. Layers of ambition bury the no-revenue-raising lessons our elders passed on to us. They do not seem supportive of our desires to advance and stay on the success track.

Harmony, kindness, generosity and fairness seem anachronisms in a corporate set-up where you wish to be a big star. So for the most part of our younger lives, we conveniently forget that, in the final analysis, we shall be measured not in terms of successes achieved or medals won but in the way we have conducted ourselves through the years – how much fun we had, how much meaning we derived from the world, how much love we shared with others. How are we to our aged parents? How are we to our children? How are we to our siblings? How are we to our remaining friends?

For a very long time, men and women validate their existences by their achievements, their career milestones, their standing in society and their possessions. As the balance sheet in the first chapter shows, these things are slowly taken away by ageing. They get reduced to digitised documents, fading photographs and mementos.

The notion that a person is ultimately measured by what he does and earns adds to the burden of ageing. People hedge at the idea of retirement, not just because they will have less money but because they are worried about the irrelevance bin to which, without their desks and accompanying paper shuffling, they will be consigned.

Couples with ego problems end up in contentious partnerships. Regular showdowns occur, spurred by the desire of one or both to prove who calls the shots. Sometimes, argument is provoked by the aggrieved party wanting to bolster self-esteem. The relationship, in this case, is a long-drawn work-in-progress. It can be a protracted contract of accommodation and concession salved, in turn, by financial security. It can even stem from nothing more than an inexplicable, gritty determination by both to see the tiring contest through to a bitter end.

Harry and Callie were married when they were in their mid-20s. They were both academics. However, just four years into the marriage, a pharmaceutical company recruited Callie and from then on things changed rapidly. At first, they both thought her very large pay packet was a big break for them. So they bought a small house and postponed having children. But it wasn't long before cracks in the relationship began to show. Callie's repeated comments about how staid and boring were their old friends annoyed and upset Harry. She also kept badgering him to be more ambitious and to look to other fields of endeavour, accusing him of being "too laid-back". They argued a lot, made up and were all right until the arguments flared up again a few months later. In the end, they turned to counselling, only to realise they were very different individuals who really didn't even like each other anymore. They were divorced soon after their eighth wedding anniversary.

When tackling relationship issues, it is helpful to review where things begin for couples. We could have got together in our 20s or 30s or 40s. We could have begun as young people wishing to explore the world together. We could have been two disillusioned individuals wanting to have another crack at happiness after recovering from failed marriages. Whatever the circumstances, the same basic requirements for nurturing relationships apply.

- **You enter a relationship as a "whole" individual, focused and centred.** By the time you commit to a partnership, you should have done a lot of reflection and settled much of the confusion and inner turmoil that may have plagued your earlier years. You shouldn't expect him/her to be your private therapist. There are limits to what our loved ones can do for us. To say someone is your rock or your anchor is not synonymous to saying he/she helps you analyse your phobias, your prejudices, and your dislike of certain cousins, your self-denials and various defence mechanisms. Love's death by tedium is often the fate of those who think a relationship will help them feel "complete".

- **You must bring into a loving friendship a degree of maturity and level-headedness.** This enables you to function as a responsible person who acknowledges that this special bond is not just about *me* or *you* or *us*. A fantasy world has its limits. No matter how magical *our* togetherness is we have to know about ATM cards, saucepans and toilet rolls. It is about *you* and *me* amid other people with their own needs, desires and agendas. It is about *us* in a world of quotidian realities, of transitions and trajectories, of brief delights and protracted sorrows.

- **To expect that the other is accountable for your personal happiness is a basic mistake.** Only you can decide whether you wish to be happy or not. You can't blame the other for your self-pity, self-denial and self-inflicted misery.

- **To believe that your love can change another person is foolhardy.** You might pay heavily for such arrogance.

THE TWO OF US

For the sake of convenience, we use the word *love*. We have been conditioned to think that in order to feel complete, fulfilled and happy, love should be present in our lives. The word is now so romanticized and mystified we could equate it with the requirement for food, air and sunlight. We need love to sustain us and inspire us; we need it to help us over hurdles and through tunnels of grief.

However, our present discussion of love must start from the premise that its meaning varies, depending on regions, cultures and even social classes. Therefore we must accept that love is a notion that gets developed and stretched to accommodate other areas of life, like children and the extended family. It is not an easy concept. As one writer said, *Man is the ideal; men are what they are.* The same thing can be said about love. Love is the ideal; loving is what it is – accommodation, compromise, understanding, tolerance. Love is a massively challenging job.

We should also bear in mind that because we ultimately live in a real world, love as practised mellows with time. Or it gets impaled on the spikes that challenge it along the way – duties, obligations and changing situations.

In the West the concept is normally perceived as the emotional attachment between two people after a period of intense attraction towards each other. A period of dating and courtship has fuelled the growth of enterprises including expensive flower arrangements, brightly wrapped chocolate boxes and fanciful candle-lit dinners. The efforts expended on all the candyfloss result in the announcement of an engagement and consequent wedding bands.

This romanticised idea of attachment has seeped into Eastern consciousness where, for centuries, the notion of love was linked to filial piety, duty to family, community and society and allegiance to the State. Loyalty passed for love. Parents took it upon themselves to determine their children's destiny. Matchmakers did brisk business; girls were betrothed to boys they hadn't even met; dowries were discussed and settled. Young people were told they would eventually get used to each other. In certain languages or dialects there is no name for love, as we understand it now. It is duty that's paramount. It's a couple's duty to obey their parents, make them proud grandparents and then spend the rest of their lives preparing their children for the world. To this day, in many Asian societies, it is taken for granted that duty to one's spouse may extend to his or her parents and siblings, a case of *look after me, look after my family* contract.

Population movements and education have drastically changed the views of recent generations. Perceptions and attitudes have evolved. Young men and women no longer accept that they should spend the rest of their lives with people they did not choose. This is a qualitative development for the better of what we now like calling a global village. Since we are each other's choice, we can talk through and work at our relationship problems in a more involved and caring – albeit sometimes combative – way.

WORKING RELATIONSHIP TEMPLATE

- There is a popular notion that good friends who fall in love with each other end up with enviable marriages or partnerships. The reasoning is, since two people know each other so well they can second-guess each other and be destined for a bright, rosy future.

- The notion that a good friendship could morph into an everlasting, loving, physical relationship has not taken into account several factors. Friends, no matter how close, no matter how dear, may not be reading from the same page all the time. Therefore, they don't necessarily develop a longing for a deeper relationship at the same time.

- By necessity, it is the yearner who initiates the transition to a joint destiny. At this point the wish to change the complexion of the friendship to a romantic relationship has to be established clearly. It is also important to gauge if the other party – the yearned-for – is not "too iffy" about the situation.

- *Never assume; never presume*. Reciprocation has to be crystal clear between comfortable friends when one indicates a wish for a shared destiny. This destiny includes physical desire, shared dreams, interwoven responsibilities and a whole new set of time-bound promises.

- There is a greater responsibility undertaken by friends when they shift gears and agree to drive through a trickier patch.

- Dear friends may constantly share opinions and laugh together. BUT they only promise to meet each other at a particular time, feed each other's pets, look after each other's plants and visit when one or the other is indisposed. Friends may empathize with each other. BUT they don't have to think about sharing a mortgage, worry about each other's monthly allowance, settle each other's grocery bills and pay for each other's prescriptions. It is easy to be in total agreement with each other when you are not expected to be responsible for each other's daily expenses. *But life should never be totally dictated by monetary concerns!* In this case, if you believe that completely, where have you been all these years?

- In other words, when two friends fall in love with each other, they change the dynamics of a comfortable association they have so far enjoyed. They risk losing all that unconditional warmth for the newly hatched excitement of knowing more about the other and having more of each other.

- It is not enough that, for 10 years, you (who may be the more enthusiastic party) have known he or she hates strawberry jam, wakes up at 10:15 am and sleeps through the weekend. **There are other things you would be called upon to understand.**

- In the transition from being friends to being lovers, one party (in this case the doubter) cannot be too far behind or the initiator too far ahead. Otherwise the gap in the understanding and adjustments required in the altered arrangements would only widen with time, causing recrimination and regret. There must exist a mutual physical attraction between the parties to make the transition easier to achieve. If this sexual tension is present, both doubter and initiator will view the relationship change from the same vantage point. (You might refer to Gerald and Jill's story that we outline on the following page.)

- It is useful to remember that the things two people bring into their friendship – the shared knowledge of backgrounds, favourite snacks, pet peeves, political bias, internal clocks and preferred reading are mutually beneficial gifts. These can nurture empathy, generosity of spirit and a willingness to assist and guide each other.

- Physical intimacy, on the other hand, often inspires puzzlement, confusion and complicates an otherwise straightforward relationship. While a man may, for years, be blind to the personal taste of his best friend, what makes him groan at her lilac pair of shoes after they've shared a bed? What makes a woman angry enough to

141

edit her erstwhile dear friend's guest list after hearing him snore, realising what a hopeless scatter bug he is and that he habitually uses his credit cards to the max?

- Would the leap into intimacy work? The awful answer is, it all depends. For instance, what was the friendship like before the shift began? Was it balanced, or was it weighed heavily in favour of one with the other constantly conceding? Was it conducted on equal terms or was one the shadow of the other? Have the two weighed the pros and cons of a changed situation?

- Having weighed all the facts, it must still be borne in mind that the established givens would change, no matter what promises are exchanged.

- Different emotions would emerge. Equally, entirely new sentiments would be aired and new demands made.

- The introduction of passion and sexuality into the picture makes fresh challenges inevitable. The gift of a shared knowledge becomes a load that has to be saved against all the new things that have to be fathomed.

Gerald, 44, and Jill, 39, went through an acrimonious divorce two years ago. A year after the separation, he quit his practice, left the city and settled on a 32-acre property in the country where, by Jill's account, he works an olive grove. Jill remains in the city, holed up in the lovely townhouse she got from the divorce. There are no children. She sees a therapist twice a week, trying to, in her words, "process all the things that happened between us and where we may have got it wrong".

They first met when Gerald was 27 and Jill was 22. He was a civil engineer and career-driven; she a trained classical pianist who occasionally taught piano to children when she wasn't on one of her trips to Europe where she enrolled for language courses or worked for a Cordon Bleu certificate.

Gerald gave most of his waking hours to his profession and could trace a time-line marking the earlier ups and downs of his career. He tackled the hard times and was rewarded by a bourgeoning career that saw him, finally, top of the class. Meanwhile, Jill – again in her own words – was "trying to find myself, pulled in various directions by many interests". There would be weeks when she was preoccupied with baking cakes or just thinking whether she should go to Tokyo to be proficient in origami, or creating a montage of pictures taken during skiing trips when she was a teenager.

They soon became very dear friends and people expected them to get married any time; an expectation that lived on year after year. Gerald and Jill were pals for 10 years. Once, they even went together with two of Gerald's friends driving across Australia's Nullarbor Plain. The trip took 11 days. As Jill recalls: "We could drive past vast stretches of desert without exchanging a cross word".

She says: "Gerald was a very good influence on me. With him as my friend, I felt more settled. He encouraged me to be more purposeful, to concentrate more on my piano proficiency and turn it into a serious practice. As he liked saying, one should have something meaningful to wake up to each day. He said I tended to fritter away my time. He said it kindly. I admired him a great deal and listened to him. So I started my children's piano workshop. I felt very good when Gerald dropped by and said, 'Well done, Jill.' He was very supportive and encouraged me to set up small piano recitals for my pupils. He was no-nonsense and was impatient with trivial matters. He was always focused at making something work. I thought he was too restless and wished sometimes he would be more relaxed. At the same time, I liked being with him.

"I initiated the seduction. We had been friends for 10 years; neither of us was getting any younger. I wanted something more permanent. I wanted my own home and I wanted him in it. At the beginning, Gerald said he wasn't too sure; he said he felt too settled in his ways and that was the thing that was making him hedge – not that he did not like the idea of us together, he added. I must admit he was, from the start, too "iffy" about the situation. But I persisted and I convinced him that nothing would change, that we should at least give it a try. I know that was foolish but I was desperate for something. I proposed. We agreed not to have children, not while we were settling in to being a couple. That was his condition."

The marriage lasted more than five years; but it didn't take a year before their comfortable friendship of 10 years deteriorated into sulks and days of silence. Jill confesses to having had anxiety attacks all the time. She so wanted to please Gerald who did not seem happy with the lovely living room and the sleek kitchen and the imaginative table setting.

"Gerald lost his temper whenever I suggested we take a short trip so he could relax. He said he could relax at home and what was the matter with me? Why was I getting contentious? I must have been very needy and demanded more attention. This irked him further. Towards the end, he accused me of always shirking responsibility and being lazy, of having been spoilt rotten. I once threatened to walk out in the middle of an argument and Gerald said, 'and where would you go, Jill, you cannot even persevere teaching ten-year-olds how to play the piano.' Which, of course, was true because once we got married I gave up the workshop. I didn't know he minded that. Gerald never said anything about it until that afternoon. Now, I know I should have been more vigilant. Only now do I recall certain lines like, 'Jill, I didn't marry you for cakes.' He said that when he came home I'd started telling him about an oven I'd seen in some glossy brochure."

It was Gerald who left the marriage but it was Jill who filed for divorce. He did not contest it. What makes Jill very sad was the way Gerald walked away from it all. There were no discussions about splitting items. He left her the townhouse and its contents. She was left with everything – albums, letters, cutlery, pictures and furniture.

Is it better if people start from a blank canvas?

If we take the example of Gerald and Jill's marriage, the answer is, yes. Yes, because with a blank canvas, there is nothing at stake; there is no gift of a shared knowledge that further intimacy might shatter, bringing disappointment, anger and misery.

Strangers who become attracted to each other are free to explore the possibilities of a relationship without the fear of wounding each other and losing the gift of shared knowledge that old friends enjoy. New acquaintances may walk through parks and go to the movies and dine together regularly for a certain period of time. They may then go their separate ways when one or both lose interest or decide there is no point pursuing something that, perhaps, is just not worth all the trouble.

The presence of sexual tension and the emotive vibes that trigger the incessant calls, the cryptic emails and the generous dinners warn new friends of the uncertainties ahead. Nevertheless, despite the occasional awkwardness, the pursuer and the pursued go through a brilliant romantic patch that – to their infatuated minds – temporarily sets them apart from the rest of mankind. The erotic excitement of being together and being buoyed by merely watching the other pour wine or struggle into a swimsuit are experiences denied old friends like Gerald and Jill.

Of course, the brilliance dims as the relationship moves on and familiarity makes them return to the normal world of bank overdrafts, office intrigues and hurrying pedestrians yelling into their mobile phones. Still, because of their "newness" to each other, the relationship is buoyed by the desire and the willingness to discover more of the other. Do we go further? Or are we now bogged down by routine? Are we good for each other?

There will be heartache if the romance is nipped by the inconsistency of one or the possessiveness of the other. Whatever the reason, the break-up could not be as gut-wrenching or as bitter as the end of Gerald's and Jill's relationship. There will be tears and the pain may be intense but recovery from love will be reached after a reasonable interval. Even minus the marriage, Jill's persistence in the shift from a long-term friendship to shared destiny and Gerald's obvious initial aversion to it already held the warnings of massive grief. His retreat to the olive grove and her being in therapy for two years are sufficient proof of this grief.

MANAGING THE TRANSITION

Whether people have been friends for years or known each other for only six months, there are some basic requirements they need to examine before they decide to be together.

- **Communication** – People skilled in articulating their feelings, thoughts, opinions and wishes to others are most likely to get the best from relationships. People are not mind readers and you must not think you can read their minds either. Drop the habit of saying "But I thought. . ." Or, "I took it for granted that she. . ." So often people use those expressions when they begin to give excuses for their failures. "But I thought they were calling us; you should have told me we were supposed to call them!" Or, "I took it for granted the bill was paid." Or, "I thought you'd posted the letter." And so on.

- **Reciprocity** – Each person must reciprocate the expression of the other's love. Both expression and reciprocation need to be established very clearly. Only afterwards can gestures be substituted and counted as expressions of love. Otherwise, it will be all presumption and assumption. The onus of making a relationship work has to be shared, which is only possible when there is mutual exchange of affection.

- **Commitment** – Both parties must recognise that their pledge to each other will, by necessity, establish reasonable restrictions on their otherwise free-wheeling life styles. These limits need to be discussed, understood and observed.

- **The value of space** - Suffocation destroys a relationship fast. While you may be committed to the partnership or the marriage, you must give each other some breathing space to retain your individual character as a human being. The insistence by one for one hundred per cent togetherness in everything could lead to the other losing his/her sense of self in the relationship. Nobody wants to be a shadow or an echo. Space can even refer to the rooms you now share. You should be mindful of each other's ways. It may be difficult for a scatter bug to learn the habit of tidiness but if he wishes to remain in the good books of Miss Neatness, he should start picking up his socks, putting back that album on the shelf and folding the newspapers after reading the sports pages.

- **Respect** – We cannot say we love or like people we treat with disdain. Living together doesn't give us the licence to own each other. It doesn't give us the freedom to intrude into the other's physical or mental space without considering his/her present preoccupations. We should not fall into the habit of demanding attention from our partners regardless of what they are doing; like telling your wife to turn off the radio programme she's listening to because you want to discuss the exorbitant airfares to London. You might argue that you are taking her on holiday – so what? It does not give you the right to be ill-mannered. Nor should we expect our partners to confess details of all their preoccupations with us. There are reasons why people may appear absent from us every now and then – it could be a work problem, a misunderstanding with a colleague or a silent budgeting exercise – and if they prefer not to discuss it with us right now, leave it be. Always keep in mind that even those who live with us are entitled to brief periods of silence to be by themselves, on their own. It is disrespectful to accuse them of disloyalty or selfishness when they are claiming this entitlement.

- **Transparency and responsibility** – If a relationship is to work and mature, partners must be broadly well informed about each other from the beginning. You should not hold back when things crop up in early conversations. If she says, "my parents expect me to dine with them occasionally", he should ask what "occasionally" means. Two Saturdays a month? Every Friday? Once in two weeks, what? If he volunteers that he enjoys poker sessions, she should ask how often does he play and how big are the games? These illustrations are given here because they could be potent spoilers to a relationship. There is, of course, an endless list of spoiler possibilities.

Accept that everyone deserves a past. How much of it do you have to share with each other? As long as it isn't likely to affect the relationship in the future, you have the right to be the sole owner of your happy secrets and you should respect the other's right to his/hers. But there are other cases that must be tabled and mutually accepted – a child by a past indiscretion, for instance, or a genetic reality in one's family, or a past nervous disorder.

Things should be clearly defined in order to avoid any "I thought you wouldn't mind" instances. If you don't ask questions, you may end up with a control freak that makes you feel it's a crime to have coffee with your father or a needy person who can't be left alone in a flat. As has been said earlier, *never assume; never presume*. Never assume that because someone has declared their undying love, they would be ready to educate your younger brother, accept your schizophrenic aunt or join your liking for tripe and reality TV shows. Never presume that because they haven't reciprocated your overtures for a bright tomorrow, they will be amenable to sharing the rent 50-50, have your cantankerous mother every weekend and happily join you in your annual Christmas boycott.

- **Financial arrangements** – Love doesn't exempt people from the tricky issue of money. You will know when the enticing segment of courtship is over when one of you turns to the other and asks, "do you have some loose change?" Or some similar question. Or when you begin discussing credit card bills. It means you have become comfortable with each other to the point that you should now be able to discuss who takes care of what. The earlier you discuss the financial side of your relationship, the better. This exercise is called apportioning responsibility. A person has to come clean and no more pretending he owns the posh flat he is renting for some astronomical price he finds difficult to pay. A woman should say whether a part of her salary goes to the maintenance of her aged parents. Nobody needs surprises in the money area. Do they pool their money together or do they retain separate accounts? How do they manage the housekeeping bills? Are there assets, like a studio flat and a portfolio of banking shares inherited from grandparents; are there liabilities, like gambling debts or children by a previous relationship? What are they willing and/or able to share?

There has to be a plan to guide the partners. Of course it must not be too rigid as to remove all the magic in the relationship. He shouldn't expect her to pay for half the candle-lit anniversary dinner and she should not charge him half the price of the shirt she bought for his birthday present. The point is, you must settle the bigger issues and be more relaxed with the small things that rekindle the attraction that brought you together in the first place.

- **A tidy mental ledger** – Relationships can last only if you are not continuously toting up points to prove you are the "better half" of the partnership. Listen to these statements: "Why am I doing all the driving?"; "How many times should I suffer your cousins?"; "I paid for all the Christmas presents between 2002 and 2006!" (Said in 2012); "I can't forget what you said about **that.**"

  While you may not forget, you must forgive if you decide to stay the course. A pile of grudges is heavy baggage to carry and it's insidious. Sooner or later it will poison your relationship. You may choose to stay together but it's doubtful whether the one carrying the load will be truthfully OK. Whatever you have forgiven, it must remain neutralised and locked away and never used as a weapon against the offender in a current and entirely different issue.

- **Acknowledgement of differences** – You can't take anything for granted because once you are together it will be difficult to sort out glaring differences. Think about these examples. Are you both early or late risers? Are you both frugal or is one a spendthrift? Do you both like socialising or is one reclusive? Do you both enjoy family life? Unless discussed, with mutually agreed compromises reached early on, a relationship between opposites is almost certain to be stormy

- **The spirit of accommodation** – No matter how many things you agree on, there will always be situations where the two of you maintain divergent views. Discuss these things as you would with friends. Forget about having the last word on everything. Learn to agree to disagree.

A SHARED DESTINY

Through the years, a couple's commitment to their relationship is bound to be tested time and time again. A partnership or a marriage remains a work-in-progress until it ends in separation or death.

No matter how close two people are, no matter how many things they agree on and no matter how brilliantly they have discussed the way they should conduct their life together, they will still experience periodic troughs. There will be threatening episodes that cause them to review attitudes towards their relationship and each other. These difficult segments are caused by various factors.

- **Increased responsibilities** – A shared life spells a host of increased responsibilities for both partners. In a two-income partnership, one option may be for the couple to pool their net salaries and then work out together how best to use and distribute their earnings. Ideally, they should keep a ledger of regular expenses, such as mortgage or rent and utility payments, insurance premiums and so on (all mostly fixed amounts) as well as savings (which may vary) and entertainment and travel costs (adjustable). After the more clinical distribution of funds the couple will need to decide how much personal allowance each needs. This, along with the entertaining and travel budget, is the tricky part, and it is here that the couple have to be prepared to listen to each other and reach decisions without conflict or unnecessary drama.

If only one partner is working, the same ledger must be kept. But the role of the partner who handles the housekeeping budget should be discussed and agreed upon. Homemaking has to be recognised as more than the duty of the person assigned to it, more often than not by default. Therefore, he/she must be entitled to a personal allowance similar to the one adopted by a two-income couple. This is an area that has often been allowed to fester over the years. Many ageing couples still nurse it as another point of dissension.

- **Children and the challenges of parenting** – Romance can fade with the appearance on the scene of a child or children. The often frantic efforts of couples to find time only for each other – rallying grandparents for babysitting, paying for a babysitter, etc – add pressure to

154

the daily requirements of working and keeping a home. Unexpected pregnancies cause a black hole in the budget and the ledger has to be reviewed and adjusted. What happens to entertaining? What happens to holidays? What about the savings? These have to be resolved. As the children grow up, life gets more complicated. Parenting attitudes towards rearing and discipline must be aligned. The awareness that *you and I* are role models to these young people we've created imposes a big sense of accountability that needs to be weighed and reviewed constantly. The boundaries on how far these children should be assisted financially should also be discussed and agreed on – this is very important.

- **Additional or changing aspirations** – We keep growing emotionally and intellectually and the fact that we are in a relationship does not change this one iota. A partner may, after 10 years of marriage, announce that he/she wants to pursue a postgraduate course. Or, after five years of togetherness, a hatred is declared for the grubby kitchen and lobby. They must be enhanced. Or, a husband may decide to quit a high-paying but soul-destroying job and start a small picture framing business. Or a wife may get a fellowship grant that would take her away for 10 months. These are testing periods to be confronted with care and compassion.

- **Major health glitches** – Health insurance premiums take care of the material part of sudden illnesses. So we should focus more on the emotional and psychological aspects.

The partner who suffers a major illness experiences a trauma that may cause clinical depression. He/she may be quieter, slower to react, become more withdrawn and reflective. It is not proper for the comparatively healthier partner to pretend nothing has happened, to keep repeating, "it's all right" – because it's not all right! – and to insist on carrying on with the usual routine. This incongruence may result in puzzlement on the part of the ill partner – "How could he/she be so constantly cheerful?" – and irritation on the part of the caregiver – "How can he/she be so self-indulgent and difficult!" This is an aspect you should discuss while the two of you are still reasonably healthy and can look at things more dispassionately. You must listen to the wishes of the other and together recognise the practicalities involved in care giving.

- **Finances** – As responsibilities increase, aspirations get revised. Health problems occur. The financial ledger will certainly require revisiting. Couples should be realistic and listen to each other when trying to resolve divergent views. Selling the large house after the children have flown the coop, cutting down on expensive travelling, whether to give the children some cash following an unexpected financial windfall, and the path of your life together when it contracts – these are the sorts of issues that call for mature handling. You are in it together. Listen to each other.

- **Extended family issues** – In later years, couples may be confronted by the changing circumstances of their extended family. Remember what we said earlier. It is not just about *me* or *you* but *us* and how *we* relate with the rest of the world. No matter how close you are and how congruent your views, your loyalty to each other can't be absolute to the exclusion of others. If you take the attitude that only the two of you matter and that each must give only the other total attention, you will find many bleak spots in your ageing years. What do extreme self-centredness and selfishness reap? These are some safe guesses: estrangement from previous working relationships, lost friendships and isolation.

Most of life is about sharing. No matter how private and reclusive you are, there must be some space given where you can contribute to the world. Of course this must, again, be arrived at after much discussion and an agreement reached without acrimony. If your wife's mother is widowed and she loses the family home, would it be OK with you to lose your guest room so she could stay with you? What could be an alternative? How would you tackle the ambitions of children by a previous marriage? How much attention would you be willing to give the problems of your brothers-in-law, your cousins and their partners? A closely-knit family has many positive sides to it but there are boundaries to keep if the goodwill is to remain.

- **Emotional issues** – There will be periods in a relationship when romance, magic and passion are absent. Routine and familiarity impale them. There will be days when you may not even like each other. There will be times when one feels hurt and resentful for being neglected and taken for granted.

Couples should always be prepared to compare notes and advise each other about what lurks as a troublesome issue. Informed, they can support each other through the biological, physiological and hormonal issues that cause puzzling mood swings. Many women who talk openly about it with their doctors and close friends hedge at discussing menopause with their partners. Likewise, men who feel a diminishing interest in sex would rather share this troubling phase with their mates. The communication gaps in such and similar instances invariably result in a great deal of misunderstanding.

Talk through your anxieties together. If you've shared a bed for 25 years, you should be able to look back on 25 years of shared victories and failures. The recipe of reciprocity, understanding and accommodation that has served you in the past should still be used beyond your productive years.

Communication may prove difficult in the fretful season of late middle age. To be dismissive, to take things for granted now, can jeopardize a relationship that has been sustained through countless challenging patches.

It is a mistake to say, "That's how she is" or "He'll come out of it" when our partners seem to be veering from the predictable course established by habit and familiarity. We should never forget that even after several decades of joint decisions, our partners remain individuals. Ageing has not stopped and should not stop them from sustaining the need for self-coherence and self-continuity which made them the "whole" persons we had been attracted to and fallen in love with.

As we age, our perceptions change and our ideas of the world are altered. These are reflected and manifested in our daily activities. The same things happen to the people we live with. We should never be dismissive of these changes – comment favourably on a positive episode and quietly bring up a discussion of an uncharacteristic negative response. Always communicate.

Every succeeding phase in human development demands the re-establishment of psychic coherence and continuity. The feelings of loss and the inconveniences that accompany the process of ageing cause periodic ruptures in an individual's sense of wholeness. The rupture caused by retirement needs to be resolved and the unpredictable emotions this phase may play out could be extremely confronting. The retiree needs patience, affection and support as he/she eases into an altered level of existence and regains congruence with different surroundings. The onset of menopause can also rupture a woman's self-esteem. She should be accorded the kindness and generosity required as she navigates her way back to wholeness.

Therefore, in a moment of helpless pique don't just say, *"You are no longer the person I married!"* Always be prepared to qualify, explain and exchange thoughts honestly. Talk through your fears, your new insecurities and the approaches you could adopt together.

- **New compromises** – Life can't remain static. Your 70-year-old wife may bring up the idea of spending more time (say, three months each year) with your son's family. A grand idea but for the fact that your son lives in Nova Scotia! But she wants to do it before rheumatoid arthritis overtakes her affection for her two grandchildren. Your husband may suddenly feel a passion for the country and, in his late 60s, express the wish to build a stone cottage. These are just two examples. Once more, involved discussions must precede every decision. Make known all your reservations and, once you have accepted the compromise, have the grace to play your part in making it happen.

- **Unexpected transitions** – As you grow older, your children and members of your extended family are also making their developmental journeys. What happens when their marriages break down, when their own children go wild, when they lose their jobs, when your 40 year-old son asks for a loan – whatever – and they turn to you? This is where you apply the boundaries you have set as a couple. Whatever assistance you give or don't give must be a joint decision and mutually acceptable to both. It is during these involved periods that you might discuss your preferences for your old age in terms of accommodation and care.

You could also start discussing the inevitable end times and what your wishes are. This is not to be treated as macabre. As you have outlined your life's trajectories in the early years, you must now face the reality that life ends sometime and you must prepare each other for this inevitability.

- **New demands on each other.** Ageing can bring out old habits and eccentricities that became dormant when we were younger, then making a living, raising children and finding our way in the world. Never lose the sense of purpose that made you interesting to one another in the earlier years. Don't form the habit of saying, now that we are retired and old, what is there to do?

Well, here's news for you. There's one purpose in life you'll have to carry through and down the years – making your shared life sustain its meaning and enhancing its riches till death do you part. This task could be as challenging as the profession or career you nursed to excellence for 35 or 40 or 50 years.

In our 60s, 70s, and 80s, we may be restored to being the youths who snacked at 2 o'clock in the morning, or loved to be read to while drinking breakfast juice, or sitting quietly on a garden bench. Your wife may suddenly develop a passion for waltzes. How do we work out sudden whims? Do we argue or do we fall in? Only the two of you can resolve this. It could be testy. It could be infuriating. It could be maddening. But a solution is there somewhere if you both decide that the present aggravation is nowhere near the big crises you've survived together.

But consider this: How old are the two of you? How long have you been together? How massive is your shared trunk of memories? And here you are – with dentures, aching joints, balding pates and ageing spots – but together.

Add this: Ageing together gives you the chance to prove what capable human beings you are – how resilient, how generous, how forgiving, how reliable, how accountable and how hopeful that, in the time left, there would still be sufficient space for fun and meaning, if you keep trying.

YOUR PHYSICAL SAFETY

Ageing couples must always keep a focus on their health and their physical safety. Hospital admissions among the elderly indicate falls as the leading cause of injury-related cases reported every year. More than half of falls occur within our homes or our immediate surroundings. Most of these slips, trips and falls are preventable and the injuries caused can be minimised. While, as we grow even older, we may "lose our bounce" or "lose the spring in our steps", we can still ensure a healthy and independent existence if we take measures in securing a safe environment for one another.

PREVENTIVE MEASURES

As we grow older, we face more risk factors – decreased muscle tone, poor balance, and bad eyesight – which can cause sprains and falls. Couples need to help each other diligently address their respective risk factors. This way they will certainly reduce the likelihood of injury.

- Be sensible and accept the limitations of age. Avoid doing multiple tasks at the one time since ageing slows down reaction times, making concentration more difficult.

- Allow for sudden changes in light levels, such as when you emerge from dim rooms into the glare of a hot day, or when you enter your dark kitchen after hours of working in your sunlit garden.

- Follow a daily exercise regimen, with focus on balance. Have your eyes checked regularly and make sure your prescription glasses are still okay.

- Don't be embarrassed to ask if you need assistance in carrying or lifting something.

- Seek the advice of a nutritionist and have a healthy diet.

- Review your home layout and if you feel you have major risk factors, seek a home safety assessment. Make sure the arrangement of furniture and accessories about your home allows for easy movement.

- Avoid poorly fitted slippers. Wear comfortable footwear with slip-resistant soles.

- Avoid wearing too loose clothes or too long dressing gowns that could catch on items.

- Have your medications reviewed regularly. Never self-medicate or take supplements without confirmation they neither contradict nor cancel benefits of prescribed medicines you've already been advised to take.

- You should keep a careful list of the medications – both prescription and non-prescription.

- Clean out your medicine cabinet regularly. Throw out unwanted or expired medications responsibly by surrendering them to your chemist.

YOUR HOME

Like ourselves, our homes do age and we may not notice the general wear and tear because we've been there for years.

It is advisable to look around the premises and see where things can be improved to make daily chores easier to handle.

- Keep frequently used areas well lit.

- Turn on lights before moving about.

- Have a torch handy all the time. It's preferable to have one on your bedside table.

- Low voltage night-lights are a good idea for passageways and corridors.

- Light switches should be easy to reach.

- Sturdy handrails should be installed in bathrooms and lavatories.

- Non-slip mats are required in the shower or bathrooms.

- A chair may help in the shower recess if you tend to be anxious.

- Take your time walking up stairs; hold on to handrails.

- If you renovate, opt for non-slip material for floors.

- If you have to get something from a higher level, don't stand on a chair. Use a proper stepladder.

- Keep walkways free and remove unnecessary cables and cords lying about. Cords and cables should be coiled and taped down next to walls or under furniture. Decorative mats and precious rugs should have slip-resistant backing.

- Rip off or repair any floor covering that is torn or

stretched. Immediately wipe up liquid spills and look out for slippery surfaces. Using contrasting tape, highlight hazards like edges on stairs and walls. Keep floor surfaces and pathways clear at all times of obstacles including your garden hose and tools. Repair cracks and check out for uneven areas in the yard outside the home.

- If you keep pets, make sure your beloved dog is not underfoot before you get moving.

- There's no need to rush. If you're feeling a bit anxious, sit back and let a few minutes pass. Rushing makes you anxious.

PRESCRIPTIONS FOR OLD LOVE

- Keep prodding each other on when you are tempted to just sit back and let the rest of life pass you by. Never use age as an excuse to ignore the changes around you. You don't have to embrace the latest technological advances but be aware they are there and what they are about. Don't alienate yourselves by being dismissive of things that don't interest you.

- Be constantly supportive of each other. Whether it is a renewed interest in dancing or a rediscovered passion for astronomy, show that it also matters to you. Sometimes, the pronouncements may only amount to a wish. Think of a couple on the porch of this house they've lived in for decades. The man says, "I wonder what it would be like to have a stone cottage in the country". The woman joins in, "A cottage with a creek behind it so you could have a beautiful view through the shrubs from the kitchen window. Then they lapse into a companionable silence. In all likelihood they would never get that stone cottage. Let us put their combined age at 144 years. But their congruence presents a happy picture.

- Constantly stoke the deep affection you have for each other. Compare how cold or how warm your hands are. Hold hands. Look in each other's eyes when you talk. When was the last time you cupped your partner's face with your hands?

- Occasionally visit your treasure trove of happy memories and again share the laughter that sustained you over the years of shared challenges. Happy remembrances make you realise the journey has been worthwhile.

- Beautiful memories should inspire you to gather more material for your memory bank. So keep sharing mutual interests and keep active together. Walk to the library. Make a couple of sandwiches and have lunch in the park. Read to each other. Visit a plant nursery together. Dig up an old recipe file and try cooking together.

- Keep nurturing old friendships. You should not allow the world to shrink into a den for two. Other points of view help the journey through old age be more meaningful.

- Have the grace to be grateful for the things you have survived so far. A thankful approach to life begets rewards. Focus on the positive side of your life together. You've journeyed this far; isn't it too late for regurgitating old hurts?

- Maintain that respect for each other's space that allowed you both time to reflect and continue to grow as complete individuals.

- Look after each other. When one is feeling down, the other must try to infuse positivity. Always remember the need for empathy.

- Never let the sun set on anger. Resolve the hurt as soon as you possibly can. Then forgive unconditionally. It's too late for mind games.

- Give time to little gestures of affection. You now have all the time to indulge each other. You don't need to go shopping for expensive gifts. In fact, the less you spend on the gesture, the better it is. At the end of each day, in bed, turn to each other and say how glad you are to be growing old together.

CHAPTER 6

THE REST OF YOUR LIFE

Don't retire!

That's sound advice. It's a good start when discussing a topic that has exercised people's minds to distraction.

It's about time we viewed the retirement issue from a certain perspective – away from farewell parties, good-bye gifts of pens, watches etc., and a grudging walk towards the sunset.

The morning after his retirement party, grumpy George asked his long-suffering wife: "Why do people insist on giving watches and pens to people who are retiring? What need do I have for a watch and a pen now that I'm not working anymore?"

But why not? They may be unimaginative going away presents, considered "safe" and unlikely to offend personal prefernces, but watches and pens likewise represent the continuation of a serviceable life where tardiness is frowned upon and the recording of thoughts remains important. Yet, people who have just been farewelled by colleagues often miss this point.

Cut off finally from desks and timetables that had validated them for years, retirees focus on the perceived loss of status and consequent irrelevance. We could tell, by his question, that grumpy George would only turn grumpier in the months ahead. He did.

Things improved but only after a long, trying period of adjustment for the whole family, including the children who had left home and started their respective families.

George's wife's recalls: "I quit working when the children were to start secondary school. George and I agreed they needed closer parental guidance and since he had just got a promotion, I opted to take leave from my nursing job. I took to full-time homemaking with gusto. The years just flew; the boys grew up, got their degrees, started working, got married and made us grandparents. Everything was OK, and then George retired. He was 65. We used to talk about it two or three years before it happened. George said we would travel and a year before his retirement, he started taking golf lessons. But when he finally retired, it was as if we hadn't discussed anything before. A stranger who nitpicked his way through the day now confronted me. Nothing was right about the house. I was wasteful and disorganised, etc. etc. He resented the time I spent chatting with my friends on the phone. He started questioning my budgeting and everyday he told me to cut down on this and that. I was getting sick of it all. It got so bad our older son invited me to stay with them for a while. I stayed away two weeks. The boys had a word with their father who didn't understand why I was getting, in his definition, "troublesome". Somebody suggested counselling. I agreed and put my foot down. If George didn't go, then I was out of there forever. Meanwhile, I was also talking my head off, whingeing about the situation."

The counselling sessions, which lasted nearly a year, had a rocky start. George initially refused to acknowledge the marriage was at a crossroads. Nina, for her part, gained in confidence and remained on her high horse. The breakthrough came when, in one of the sessions, their older son said, "I know it's a very difficult time but I believe we can solve our problems. Despite everything, I'm sure my parents really love each other."

George and Nina were taken aback and when the therapist asked – "Do you agree with what your son just said?" – George replied, without hesitation, "*Of course*". Nina nodded, but couldn't speak . . . because she had started crying.

Gradually, George and Nina were able to work out a plan where they could stay together without getting on each other's nerves. He realised he was wrong simply barging into what used to be Nina's domain, criticising things he had overlooked or dismissed as "not so important" in the years when he felt "important" outside the home. Did it really matter how she organised the pots and pans? Did her choice of curtains make her inept? How could she become an incompetent homemaker overnight? Nina, for her part, began to understand that the man who had been "paying for everything" was "a changed man" because retirement made him feel "unmoored" and therefore "lost at sea".

At 66, George began his volunteer work in a local hospital. Once a week, he called on two or three cancer patients needing radiation and drove them to the hospital. During their treatment he had coffee with the acquaintances who had introduced him to the programme. Soon, he took on other tasks. He offered to cook dinner twice a week, which Nina welcomed. He had long wanted to learn another language and so decided to do something about it. He thoroughly enjoyed the Spanish course, creating new friendships. When he was feeling truly relaxed about his new schedule, he was called for consultancy work in his old company. They needed two retirees to do part-time mentoring. George was offered three days a week, and opted for two.

By the time he turned 68, George felt very comfortable with his "new life". He's still doing the mentoring job twice a week. He says he wishes he had been given the same training benefits when he was navigating himself through the workforce. Life would have been easier, George believes, if he had been guided through time management and prioritising interests.

This is what he now says: "I tell the young men and women I mentor that while they must be vigilant and devoted to their jobs, they must remember they also have lives beyond work. They need to learn how to apportion their precious time so that nothing or no-one gets neglected. It can be done. A lot of people do what I once did. I used my job as an excuse to stay away from things I considered trivial or boring and that sometimes included family activities. I watch my sons with their children and I see what I've missed."

For 45 years, George had been employed by corporations, going up the career ladder each time he changed jobs. In the last 20 years he had become used to a ritual where his existence was validated by his name plastered on a door and a desk. He had a private secretary. From this tiny fiefdom, he dispatched and answered letters, took part in telephone conferences and worked himself through many office intrigues. Work was his world. His job defined him.

As his retirement loomed, George would discuss the future with Nina. Looking back, he recalled all they used to talk about at length, but their conversations were at best "sketchy".

So when George retired, he took for granted he could, without preliminaries, seize and control Nina's long-held territory.

WORRYING IS NOT PLANNING

Many people nearing retirement are like George. They worry about how life will be as a retiree and talk a lot about it. *Will they get bored? Will friends remember them? Will the nest egg be sufficient?* They regurgitate these conversations until they get to believe they are preparing for retirement. They talk about "plans" – trips with their families, re-location, a new hobby – but often these only constitute a list of intentions and are never properly fleshed out.

Planning for retirement entails a re-examination of how the past years have been and how all the free hours in the future will impact on the people previously considered "in the way" of one's jobs. Men, especially, get surprised when their awkward – and invariably annoying – attempts at asserting themselves in the home after years of emotional and psychological absence are met by either hostility or indifference. They fail to see that in the intervening years their wives have fashioned separate lives and created their own pockets of happiness which, by necessity, left their busy husbands out. Men are startled to realise the children are now grown up and their interests don't always include the "oldies".

Many people blunder into their retirement full of illusory ideas which, when punctured, bring more stress and unease.

DON'T FALL FOR THESE ILLUSORY IDEAS

1. Golf, gardening, listening to music and long lunches will be sufficient to replace decades of coping at work.

What do people say when the topic of retirement is brought up?

"About time I had time for me."

"All my life I've answered the beat of other people's drums. It will be great to dance to my own music."

"No more memos! I will wake up and the whole day will be for self-expression."

"It will be good to have the nose away from the grindstone."

"The golf course beckons!"

"Now I can concentrate on all the things I've been wanting to do."

"It will be wonderful to play life by ear."

"Spontaneity will be the name of the game once I'm out of that dungeon."

"Life will be more straightforward and simple."

When applied to retirement, these statements are illusory. If we don't have a solid game plan and depend entirely on spontaneity, retirement will be akin to stepping into a void, a catastrophic development after years and years of having defined ourselves by our salaried jobs.

Usually, such sentiments are expressed when the spectre of retirement is still a few years away. They may well be mantras people use to allay the fears of yet another challenging transition, or continuing to work at jobs that, by and large, they dislike. That being so, they are truly looking forward to endless days of self-expression and spontaneity. However, in this instance they fall into the trap of unrealistic expectations, believing their retirement will transform them into more purposeful people. The danger is they become obsessive to the point their plans form an escape from their sense of emptiness and their hopes are turned into fantasies.

Planning for retirement has to be anchored at realistic levels and must always be constructive. Many factors should be considered in planning future projects – financial position, base support (the quality of present relationships), health (physical and emotional) and other people's plans. There's no point putting a trip to Antarctica at the top of the list when you are still paying your mortgage. Taking your wife on a dream cruise along the Rhine may be tempting fate if the two of you haven't sorted out your yelling matches. It would be advisable to have a few weeks break in a quiet cottage somewhere if you are feeling exhausted or fragile. Listen to what your spouse or children are saying, which should guide you when plotting the future.

Felix, 73, volunteers: "I hated being a salesman but stuck it out because it provided well for my family and I wanted to play safe. I never felt like learning a new trade and doing something different. When I got to be sales director of the company, I thought, well, this is okay. My wife retired from teaching when she turned 55 and from then on went on a yearly trip with two or three of her friends. By that time our two children had left home. I retired at 60. My wife and I decided to go on a two-month tour of the United States, visiting family and old friends along the way. We went just a week after I stopped working. It was the most expensive, most exhausting and most disappointing journey I've ever taken. I wasn't ready for it. I should have waited until I was settled in a new routine. It was my fault entirely. I'd wanted to do something straightaway."

Felix was right. He should have given himself time "to settle". Retirement from a job that has taken much of one's life for many years to a new unchartered territory is a huge transition. While there could be buoyancy in the thought that one is "free at last", there could also be an opposing downward pull that comes every time a big chapter in one's life ends. Retirement from a full-time occupation requires a "mourning period" when the retiree has to integrate past and present so he can get on with life as realistically as possible. The time limit on this task depends on one's congruence and self-awareness.

For a great part of our adult lives, full-time employment dominates. If we are self-employed, our enterprises can even take over our lives. When retirement is foisted on us, whether by choice or circumstance, will the sweeping pronouncements made by would-be retirees – endless golf, playing life by ear, day-to-day spontaneity – be sufficient to provide the same sense of fulfilment as an honest day's work? Finding a replacement for the long hours of analysing documents, writing proposals, working out sums, sitting at meetings and meeting deadlines is a complex task. Whether you've worked with love or under sufferance becomes irrelevant when the rushing and the coping are over.

Many retirees get involved in a multitude of activities and enjoy boasting that they've never been so busy in their lives. In most cases, activity is again being mistaken for achievement. In an effort to prove that they haven't lost stature and haven't been "downgraded", many new retirees get tempted to say yes to everything. Fear seizes them when they confront the hours left vacant. They are, for instance, no longer expected to get up early, commute, rush through pending work, argue with colleagues and worry about the next big project.

Long before you retire, you should begin preparing a replacement portfolio to plug into the sinkhole when full-time work ceases. This will constitute new "work". The activities in this new folder have to be a healthy mix of constructive work and hobbies, or small interests that used to play second fiddle to "old work".

What is constructive work? Whether paid or unpaid, it should leave us feeling fulfilled or still useful. Retirees who have not thought of these constructive endeavours usually, by default, end up participating actively in the lives of their grandchildren. They may protest and complain about their schedules being stretched but in reality they are grateful for the opportunity to be "serviceable" and therefore "still visible".

Other options include going back to university as a mature student, doing consultancy work, enrolling (and finishing) courses in calligraphy or horticulture or languages, resuming musical interests, learning sign language and doing disciplined community service work. Other examples could be extensions of your old skills, or new choices, tapping your hidden talents. This may take time to firm up as new "work". If you are one of those who has always felt there's a book, a painting or a play in you, retirement may be a good time to put it to the test.

2. *Life will be a breeze.*

The end of full-time employment means you now have the choice of waking up at 6am or at mid-day. Finances permitting, you can also play tennis from dawn to dusk or depart on an extended sea cruise.

But there are other things that will first need your attention. Since there is no longer a corporation to back you up, your health insurance will be for you to either renew or let lapse. If you've driven a company car, you will have to look for new arrangements. Whatever the alternative is your responsibility – its maintenance, its insurance, and its yearly registration. You will now be responsible for your snail mail and your email, your files and folders, your address book and all your telephone calls. No more secretary or junior clerks to screen your calls and lie that you are "in conference".

3. *I will have so much time to get together with old friends.*

You may have forgotten something. Where are these friends? In the years when you were too busy, how much time did you give old friends? If you were given names of ten "old friends", would you be able to say that you know their exact whereabouts, their contact numbers and how they've been keeping the past year or so?

As we've described earlier in the book, working people tend to think that their social circle is fine because of the colleagues who surround them. After all there were all those numerous celebrations everyone enjoyed. Many old friends remain in the memory. Over the years, however, they may have moved to other states or provinces. Some may have even migrated to other countries. One or two may have died.

There is another aspect of old-friendships. Unless you've been in touch regularly over the years, meeting up with old friends – *only upon retirement, when "we finally get the time"* – can lead to disappointment. As we grow and change, other people also grow and change. We all become different individuals and expecting our old pals to have stayed as we remember them is never a good idea.

There are advantages to cultivating new friendships outside one's work environment. Count yourself blessed if, years before retirement, you have a handful of new friends, young and old. They will save you from being the sorry figure killing time at Reception until former colleagues leave their desks for lunch. Start believing you cannot regurgitate stories about office intrigues forever.

4. *The spouse and I will have lots and lots of quality time together.*

While you may have discussed the fact that you'll be home most of the time, have you imagined what your spouse will feel about the whole thing? Have you listened to what she's got to say? Have you examined the trajectories of your life together thus far? What has been your idea of togetherness?

Here's a quote attributed to the New York-based clinical social worker and therapist, Ella Harris: *A retired husband is often a wife's full-time job.*

Many retirees are unprepared for the impatience and irritation their constant presence in the home appears to generate. This can go on for months and cause considerable tension between spouses.

A man with no office to drive to or deadlines to keep will now have time to focus on many things he previously had chosen to ignore. Like George in the beginning of this chapter, a male retiree can now pad about the home that, for the longest time, has been the responsibility of his wife (this is often the case even if she's working). Like an officious inspector, he begins asking questions or passing judgements on the quality of *her* housekeeping. The kitchen cupboards are a mess. The garbage bins should be somewhere else. Do they really need fresh flowers in the living room? The curtains in the guest room are hideous. Is *this* really how she files the bills? And so on.

Years of productive interaction outside the home can easily bloat a person's idea of self-importance and sense of entitlement. Despite his good intentions, a man who retires will have to channel his need to remain feeling useful, serviceable and in control. In seeking "new territory" he will run the risk of losing boundaries. He will try to fill the void where his magnificent office once stood and where his protective secretary used to screen his calls, including those from his wife. In this case, the home will become a substitute and who do you suppose will become the secretary? So, on top of passing judgement on how the kitchen is organised, the bills are filed and the state of the curtains, he may expect his wife to manage the address book and field a few telephone calls on his behalf.

It is natural such behaviour elicits annoyance and impatience from the person who interprets these developments as unwarranted invasions of a previously uncontested landscape.

It is important for the retiree to remember that previous patterns and expectations do not change overnight. Here, then, adjustments in approach and attitude have to be made.

Spouses must discuss this part of their ongoing journey and seek a common ground from which they can move forward with renewed vigour. They need to re-examine their expectations of each other and how things will work in the midst of changed circumstances.

Months before he retired, Owen discussed with his wife the possibility of converting one of their two guest rooms – which used to be their children's bedrooms – into his home office. He had decided to do freelance copywriting and book editing. Grace readily agreed and became so enthusiastic about it, Owen said later, he was almost convinced it had been her idea. Owen always had a job that entailed a lot of travelling. Grace had never worked in her life. Having the home office ready for occupancy when Owen retired helped a great deal when the two of them were navigating their way through the new schedule after 42 years of marriage.

5. *I've got a financial adviser. I'll leave everything in his hands and just enjoy myself.*

Unless you wish to enjoy yourself to the brink of penury, you should always understand the direction your financial chart is going. You need not – should not – be obsessive but a regular review of where you stand financially is required. Your financial adviser can only lay cards on the table; the deal is yours to decide. Your decision has to be an informed one and if you are not aware of what's happening out there, how can you protect your nest egg? Remain alert and vigilant. Read. Make it difficult for other people to test your vulnerability.

REVISIONING PERSPECTIVES

Mind-sets are traps that often deny us the lessons and pleasures of changed circumstances. We get conditioned to an existence of accepted roles and habits and the rewards these bring. We form habits and nurse expectations that are difficult to dislodge because of our own refusal to adjust and let go.

Our everyday stresses are caused by the way we resist and respond to the little, sometimes even imperceptible, changes that occur around us. Our responses are shaped by our upbringing, our earlier experiences of acceptance and rejection and our learned prejudices.

We have long been conditioned to think that the end of one's working life – retirement – is virtually the end of active, useful life. Self-awareness and a healthy self-esteem should remind us that we don't have to be paid to remain contributors to society.

Congruence should make us see the promise in every transition – we retire from something (a job, a career, a profession) but we retire to something else (volunteer work, a hobby farm, a library of unread books, a hardly used kitchen, a wilderness of a garden – the options are endless).

BRIDGE JOBS

Cultivating other profitable interests outside your old, full-time work while preparing for retirement pays dividends. For purposes of convenience, we shall refer to these as "bridge jobs".

A bridge job brings us the following benefits:

- As it continues to engage us, we gain more objectivity when we view the retirement issue;

- The detachment enables us to shake off fear and trepidation;

- Freed of anxiety, the mind arrives at a well-thought out plan;

- The social interaction is a morale-booster;

- It assures us that life goes on after retirement.

When considering bridge jobs, be guided by what usually made you feel good in the past – interests or hobbies that left you feeling you'd achieved something. Generally, bridge jobs should not call for a radical re-invention; they are supposed to guide you through a huge transition from validating full-time work to a fresh existence with more free hours to fill.

The example of Victor in Chapter 1 is worth repeating here. At 47, he got into a panic mode because of retrenchment anxiety. He didn't lose his job then but the sleepless nights made him consider options other than his middle management status at the bank. He began exploring the idea of a gardening maintenance business with his sons. The small weekend transactions made his later transition from a neck-tied, desk-bound executive to a relaxed entrepreneur who decided his own schedule with considerable ease.

Tanya's return to an old interest

Tanya celebrated her 45th birthday in Shanghai. It was a childhood dream. Whether the city met her expectations or not is beside the point. What matters here is that it was in Shanghai, at a silk store, that Tanya had a panic attack.

"I was deciding between a jade green shirt and a pink one when I felt wobbly," recalls Tanya. "I went back to the hotel and rested. But I couldn't get out of my mind the possibility that I might have lost all my advertising accounts when I returned home. My career in advertising would be over. It's good it happened on the penultimate day of my holiday. I couldn't wait to get home."

All her life Tanya prided herself in being a "workaholic". She also enjoyed being referred to as being "hard-boiled" and "competitive", character traits she considered essential in an advertising career.

"I was so immersed in my career. I was so shaken by that China episode," Tanya pursues. "Prior to that my friends occasionally remarked how the years seemed to be moving faster than ever. It sounds silly now but for a long while I felt apart from all talk of time's passage. I was too busy. I had important accounts to handle and was forever pitching for new ones. I couldn't be bothered indulging in what I thought was small talk."

After Shanghai, Tanya saw she wasn't immune to the changes around her. She began noticing that younger and younger people sat at the desks in her office. She began to pay more attention to conversations about the future.

Retirement thoughts didn't come easy to her. Twice divorced, she had a son at medical school and was used to having "good things". Tanya went through a period of sometimes discussing retirement in a fragmentary, desultory manner and sometimes talking about it intensively and excessively. She found herself often distracted and it troubled her that for the first time in her stellar, high-flying job she wasn't focused. She also noticed she often found herself down in the dumps despite the regular shopping sprees. She tired easily.

Fortunately, Tanya had, over the years, gathered a few old mentors from whom she sought advice during troubled periods. This time she had long talks with the family's retired GP. She opened up and spoke openly about her sadness and her doubts about the future.

It was the GP who reminded Tanya about her earlier classical piano training. She could have gone on pursuing a career in music had the lure of big bucks in advertising not distracted her.

The upshot was Tanya started playing the piano more assiduously again. She also re-connected with old friends. One of them asked her whether she could, for a fee and when she was free, play second piano for students preparing for their junior recitals. She accepted and the occasional second piano engagement became a bright feature of Tanya's life at weekends. Consequently, she shopped less. She stopped fretting about having to leave advertising. By the time she retired at 50, she had got together with three other friends and was set on launching a small private music school.

Locum work for Kevin

The land was a major factor in Kevin's early years. He never forgot that the farming life had given him a comfortable childhood and paid for his education. He liked to recall boyhood memories of lengthy mealtimes in the farm's courtyard. The images were still vividly clear of his father sitting at the head of the table, the carafes of wine and his mother's excellent roast dinners.

Kevin loved his work as a surgeon but he was always mindful it couldn't last forever. Every now and then he would point this out to his wife and three children.

"I've always been aware of ageing," Kevin says. "My father worked the land very competently but I watched him slow down and had long conversations with him about it – especially after my mother died. I decided my practice as a city surgeon should end by the time I turned 55.

"I've talked about my retirement plans with my family for years. My wife, who's a year younger, thought 55 was too young to leave a profession I obviously loved. We discussed this ad nauseam. I told my children that I would finance their university courses but if they wished to further their studies or go overseas, they'd have to support themselves.

"My ultimate goal was to return to country life. My wife knew this from day one. She's an accountant, city-born and bred but was open to the idea of eventually moving to the country.

"I set my retirement plan early. We made regular trips to my father's old farm, which my younger brother was now running. My wife decided to do freelance bookkeeping from home shortly after our youngest child moved out. I did not wait until I was 55. When I was 53, I gave up my city practice, sold the house and signed up to do locum work in rural areas. The money was very good and wherever we went and stayed for two or three months, my wife found opportunities for doing community service. It was a great way to see the country. In between jobs we stayed in a rented cottage on the edge of the farm where I grew up. I rediscovered my siblings and renewed the friendships of the mates who had not been seduced by city lights.

"I was 58 when the locum work started to tire me. Before I turned 60, we found a beautifully reconverted barn that came with 17 acres of land, near the old property. My wife loved it instantly. Since then she has become a keen gardener and even the children can't tempt her to spend a few days with them. We've done a lot of driving; now people have to see us.

"Every now and then the town doctor goes on holiday and asks me to mind his shop. Two other friends and I go fishing regularly. My wife has a couple of bookkeeping accounts. She does volunteer work, helping out with shopping and driving for parents with disabled children.

"I am 67 now, my wife is 66. For her 65th last year, we went to visit her siblings who'd migrated to Canada. She had a fantastic time and so did I. I think we've had a good life. But it's been good only because we've always planned and have never taken things for granted."

ALWAYS LOOK AROUND

Make use of your other skills or hidden talents when thinking of a bridge job. Don't wait for opportunity to knock on your door – look for it.

Are you a linguist? Christine started giving private French classes (to groups of no more than four at a time) four years before she quit her public school teaching job at 55.

Have you had a penchant for the arts? Richard signed up to conduct summer calligraphy classes at the local community centre two years before he retired at 60. After retirement, he was invited by the community college to continue managing some courses.

Use your kitchen. Therese found working in insurance was getting her down after 25 years and began thinking of taking early retirement. She was a very good cook. She invested part of her savings in a Cordon Bleu course, travelled through Europe and when she came back registered a catering business, limiting her services to small private functions. Her first commission was to feed the board members of her insurance company. Therese took early retirement when she was 52. The bridge job grew and grew. Fortunately, she was able to share her commitments with a sister-in-law and several relatives.

Make use of what you already have. Three years before Tom retired at 65, he started supplying seedlings regularly to five gardening outlets. The seedlings came in little black plastic pots he had saved over the years. Tom had green fingers and his large garden was his joy. When he and his wife – she didn't work – were discussing his retirement plans, she suggested he should start exploring how to make the garden work financially. It took a while for the idea to germinate. His wife made the initial approaches. The venture began with small tray orders and grew from there. Tom started to sell small palms, agave, flowering plants and an assortment of herbs. A section of his garden was devoted to cultivating orchids and, by the time he retired, Tom was ready to open at weekends and sell rare breeds to orchid fanciers.

There are many other options for those prepared to engage in positive approaches to ageing and retirement. The world has its way of rewarding those who reject the notion that the heavens will simply open up and shower them with blessings. The idea is to remain resilient, open and alert.

CHARTING THE FUTURE

- Most people work until they reach the compulsory age of retirement, currently set at 65. However, a combination of factors, including financial pressures on national economies and increases in life expectancy, is likely to extend the official "working life" beyond 65 to 66 and 67. This could mean waiting another two years for their pension for those people who have already put in more than 40 years of solid work and paid taxes since they were in their twenties. Understandably, this will cause some resentment.

Certainly there are already exceptional examples of employment extended to 70 years, often for devoted academics who stay on teaching despite becoming physically slower in the hallowed halls of learning. This is fine, but the journey has to end sometime – so what may happen then? Truth is people will be better off to have their retirement plans well in place, even when they decide to extend their working life by a few more years.

Many men and women opt to be their own bosses, working doubly hard to make their enterprises grow. These self-employed people don't have the safety net enjoyed by corporation employees – if they are slack they get no income. They pay for their failures. So they work doubly hard and have less time for leisure. Retirement for enterprising men and women is determined by several factors: how much success they achieve and when, how complex their enterprise becomes (if it gets too big, it may need the injection of more capital), selling out might be a tempting option, then tiredness, of course, can be the determinant factor. Some retire at 45, some at 80.

Some occupations are more "time-sensitive", like sports. One cannot hope to be a professional player for two decades, considering all the injuries sports people suffer in the course of their careers. Players are lucky if they get to compete into their late 30s. Afterwards they have to re-invent themselves as coaches, sports commentators, newspaper columnists or online bloggers. Stars should plan their futures from the moment they start earning big money from playing and sponsorship endorsements. By all indications they should be able to build nest eggs faster than, for instance, middle management executives.

Of course, not everyone ends up a multi-millionaire from kicking a ball or punching another boxer senseless. Lesser lights are advised to think of learning another trade while they indulge their passion. Ronald is a case in point. While waiting to be the next David Beckham, he trained to be a tree lopper and ended up running a very successful tree maintenance business. Many lacklustre careers have been the seeds of flourishing enterprises like sports shops, coffee bars (within earshot of gyms) and training venues. There are builders, auto-mechanics, bookkeepers, bricklayers, plumbers and plasterers who once played basketball, rugby, soccer or another of the football versions as a full time occupation. There's also the odd doctor, scientist and lawyer as well.

The same counsel applies to actors and dancers – they have to consider the future while their careers are bright. How might they re-invent themselves as they grow older and less agile? They could become coaches, directors or producers. Those whose careers hardly take off should consider other options. They could become production assistants, dressers, set designers, teachers or even agents.

- Whatever the occupation and whatever the retirement age, there is a commonality in all the aspects we've just discussed – your financial security. You shouldn't rely completely on the government, your children or even the prospect of an inheritance.

- The middle years, the fretful period of one's life when incongruence and unresolved issues are often salved by heady careers and a sense of "runaway prosperity", could lull anyone into a costly complacency, making planning for retirement a more complex task. A sense of runaway prosperity has made countless people reckless – settling on huge home mortgages, bribing their wives or children with sports cars or dream trips to make up for neglect or misdemeanour, "investing" in horses and magnificent boats and, even when travelling privately, flying business class.

The rule is: If the full payment on the big extra is totally dependent on your salary or bonuses, don't sign the cheque. Unintelligent spending in midlife can create major hurdles if you're considering retirement.

Victor relates: "I was carried away by my mid-life prosperity. I was a risk management executive in a big bank. I earned big bucks and started thinking big. My wife wanted a sports car so I bought her one. My children went for all the lessons they could think of – ballet, tennis, riding. I gave my older daughter a horse for her

16th birthday. My wife thought of and booked expensive family holidays. She entertained often and lavishly. She liked saying she was proud of our home. She had to be – it was large and expensively furnished. For a long, heady period, I let the gravy train roll on and on. It was only after the girls were finished with university and left home that I started thinking. I had to. The bank was going through monstrous re-structuring and was no longer one of the brass upstarts. I was getting tired, too, but realised my projected retirement had to be postponed. Even with major adjustments like selling the house, downsizing and refusing to buy a replacement sports car, I had to work another five years.

"When I look back now, I realise that very little of that time made me truly happy or even content and interested. I spent and spent to keep the peace. To this day, I wonder what lessons and values we passed on to our daughters. They are reasonable children but their sense of entitlement sometimes gets out of whack. Every now and then they get in touch with their mother and drop hints about some fancy side table they dearly want locally. My wife feels it's her maternal duty to pay the freight charges. I put my foot down. Of course, consternation follows. Somehow it would appear I'm still expected to spend to keep the peace."

- Leave a margin for unexpected developments or exigencies in your retirement budget. Governments are notorious for dreaming up additional taxes. You have to shoulder the gaps in fees lodged with your private health insurers. If you intend maintaining bank overdrafts, credit cards and club memberships, keep in mind that currency and interest rates fluctuate.

- Bear in mind that the figures you enter in your retirement list are not cast in stone. The approximate sums will vary from year to year. Allow for inflation and the likely volatility of the currency you're working with.

- If you are considering spending part of your retirement funds to take over a small business – like a sandwich stall or a small antiques shop – because you wish to keep busy, think again. Nobody goes into business just to keep busy. A business has to make a profit to be worthwhile. At very least it should break even. Also, are you willing to work harder than you ever did when you were a salaried employee? How much do you know of the business you have in mind? If you claim "a lot" and that it is your "passion", then decide how much you are willing to lose for your passion every week, every month, and for how long?

- You must reach an understanding with your family – spouse and all your children – about the boundaries of their expectations. They should not expect you to: fund their graduate studies; pay for the elitist education they wish for their children; contribute funds in aid of ballet or tennis lessons; shoulder the costs of their divorces or be their Day Care Centre. You will be retired. You want to have extra time on your own. You have only sufficient funds for yourself, which, in all likelihood, you may have to stretch.

About helping your children: If you have them, you'll be parents forever. One of the unexpected demands that could rattle you in your retirement may involve your children. One of them may suddenly turn up at your doorstep with two children in tow to announce a separation from an abusive relationship. Of course you'll assist and give her temporary shelter. But your help must have its limits. It shouldn't be a rescue effort – not a good idea. While she's waiting to have things sorted out, you must help empower her. You won't be doing her a favour if you assume her responsibilities. If she's working, how has she organised the care of her children? She should continue with those arrangements or look for alternatives. You mustn't take over her life because you are a parent – that would be a disservice.

Another point about money: don't be sweet-talked into selling the family home by any of your children or relatives and moving into that granny flat above *their* carport. Even if you are considered frail and prone to colds – this would surely be pointed out to you – stand your ground. It should motivate you to look after yourself better and cultivate healthier habits.

- Include in your plan definite time-frames for your physical, mental and emotional wellbeing. This should be an everyday thing. Before starting a new physical exercise routine, consult your GP. Remain curious and alert – take the trouble to know what's happening in your midst. Try to be more open to innovation or changes. Don't allow yourself to be so cross and worked up about things that aren't to your liking.

- Make technology work for you. In your retirement, reach out to friends and family without spending a fortune. Don't say, "I'm an old retiree, I don't want to know about email and Skype." Start learning now. There's nothing wrong with technological advances as long as you are in control and don't allow them to be a substitute for actual life.

  Become a member of your local library if you aren't already. Read. Exchange ideas and opinions with others. Continue to listen.

  Do volunteer work not just to kill time but to help the community become better. It is never too late to practise some altruism. One sure way of staying on cue is to be interested. Engage regularly in activities that involve other people. Contribute ideas. Participate in discussions.

- In your retirement plan, give space for a regular review of the way you perceive the world. The self-awareness you worked hard to achieve in your middle years will continue to be challenged as life goes on. In order to remain congruent always be mindful of your boundaries and your sense of entitlement. The fact that you've lived longer and are retired does not give you the right to be acerbic, insulting and discourteous to others. Some people say, "I'm old, I can say what I want." Are they saying that we, the old, have no use for courtesy and civility?

MAKING A TRANQUIL RETIREMENT

- *Health is important.* No doubt illness can strike the body at any time, but if you have cultivated a mature attitude towards adverse circumstances, you will be in a better position to heal. A vibrant mind is a gift that should keep ticking – nourish it daily. You must keep active. Too often, people lapse into "learned disabilities". A man may feel some pain in his knee and immediately move his sleeping quarters to the ground floor so he doesn't have to negotiate a flight of stairs. Another person may occasionally feel dizzy when standing by a hot stove and give up cooking. There are also those who practise selective hearing or play at forgetfulness. Things have a way of becoming habits and these people can end up truly deaf and infuriatingly forgetful.

As we said earlier you should always have a back-up plan if your health doesn't hold. This must be in place and all the people involved in it – your spouse, your eldest son, your general practitioner, and your best friend – must be properly briefed.

- *A sense of purpose can lighten the day.* You'll feel uneasy walking around wondering what to do and ultimately ending up wasting time going around in circles. If you wake up in the morning thinking – "Before it gets too hot, I should be working in the garden", or, "I should be sorting out this month's receipts." – you are onto a good thing. They are simple chores that yield actual achievements. They leave you feeling good in yourself – the garden ends up tidy or the receipt file is updated.

- *Discipline.* Just because you are retired doesn't mean you can waste time or allow other people to waste yours. While you may need a purpose to your day, you should not settle for just any activity foisted on you by someone who wants to kill time with company. Better to stay in and listen to some soothing music than feel half-hearted while sipping a cup of overpriced cappuccino.

Know and observe your boundaries. Stick to your words and honour your promise. If, for some reason you fail, own up. This sense of ownership stops the mind flitting from one possible excuse to another. It also gives you a sense of community and makes you stay connected. If others observe that you remain respectful of your environment, are still accountable and responsible for what you say and do, they will set you apart as a role model – someone who has not been cowed by age and life.

- *Financial independence.* There's discipline needed here. too. Whether you have too much, just sufficient or too little, your purse strings must be in your control. Signing away your responsibility over your own money because you are too sickly, too lazy or too scared of machines should not be an option. You don't want to be in a position where you request your son or daughter to give you some of your money because you want to buy a new air conditioner.

  Having your financial independence feeds your self-esteem. The decisions you make regarding your assets may sometimes exercise you but ultimately they leave you empowered.

  Be prepared to make adjustments to your lifestyle if your bank balance warrants them. Even this may annoy you initially, but the whole rigmarole of what to cut and what to retain should make you feel sharp, able and in command.

- *The requirement for a good support base.* All the years of being a good parent/sibling/relative/friend should yield their dividends. In your retirement you should be able to count on sharing ideas, reflections and opinions with those whose friendships you nurtured over a lifetime.

Old friendships are one of the magical gifts reserved for the ageing.

- *A continuing interest in life.* The present may be very different from the world to which you were born. This is for the better. For every fault that leaves you aggravated, consider an opposing frame. If the world had not moved from how it was when you were born, we would still be travelling with health certificates clearing us of smallpox and yellow fever. We would still have countless men and women dying of consumption in sanatoriums. We would not be hopeful for new and better treatments for diabetes and cancer. We would have no idea of what the moon's surface is like.

  As a retiree with ample time on your hands, you can look in depth into the study of people, events and milestones. You can choose a subject and start a personal research project. Then you'll have something to talk about other than your arthritis and how much you lost on the stock market and how awful the young are these days.

- *Have more dreams than regrets.* Dreams are essential in the meaning-making process that ensures life meaningful at any given stage. The dreams and hopes we had as children, as teenagers, as young adults starting out in the world and as middle-aged individuals toiling away, kept us going. There's no reason why, in retirement, we should stop envisioning a future where we see ourselves at peace with the world and ourselves.

- *Sharpen your sense of thankfulness.* Rather than wallow in sadness when recalling happy events, think instead of how privileged you've been having experienced them. Be glad they happened. Consider the luck you've had in having come this far, in having lived through both blessings and hurdles. How else can you show your gratitude? Make each day count by trying to inject meaning into it. Just enjoying yourself is enough.

- *Practise kindness daily.* It is easy to find fault and very easy to deliver angry speeches that cut people down. Kindness goes a long way in making others feel positively disposed towards you. This does not mean you shouldn't register displeasure if they've erred. But you can say your piece without verbally lacerating the offenders. If you wish for an old age of desolate isolation where people tiptoe about you and say only what they think you want to hear, cruel words pave the shortest route to it.

- *While you may be making adjustments to your financial chart, don't stop treating yourself altogether.* You may have to forego the big overseas trip this year or buying the luxury car, but it shouldn't drive you into a big sulk. Challenging financial times test character. Use your imagination. If the expansive things you've done in the past were done for your pleasure and not to impress others, pursuing scaled down activities shouldn't be difficult. All too often, people refuse to adapt to changed circumstances because they worry about other people's opinions. You should be past this now.

- *Occasionally surprise your spouse.* One afternoon, when his wife Jenny was visiting a sick friend in hospital, Keith, 76, watched Jamie Oliver on television and took down notes. He had never cooked before. Jenny returned home in the early evening. Understandably, she was rather depressed and tired. But Keith had the oven humming and some vegetables blanching. Jenny was overwhelmed. The simple gesture lifted her spirits.

- *Tidying.* Start tidying your surroundings by doing away with insignificant clutter. Chances are you have piles of group snapshots with people whose names you can't even recall taken at events that no longer register. Keep only photographs that still hold emotional meaning and are therefore relevant to your present. There are batches of souvenirs gathering dust in cupboards. There are pictures you no longer like still hanging on your walls. They are items you bought on impulse, exiled in various nooks, and you hate them. There are two old Christmas trees that have sat in the garage for a decade. There are old shirts, trousers, ties and belts, never to be used again because they are now a couple of sizes smaller, still crowding your wardrobes.

Retirement is the excellent time to do away with the mistakes, the unwanted and the meaningless. Learn to let go. Keep on weeding pruning, and re-organising.

Then one day you'll wake up to rooms where you'll be surrounded only by things that define you. Having done away with so much clutter you may just be convinced, finally, that one only has to simplify life to make its significance shine through.

Life will go on and it won't matter whether you're 75, 80 or even 90 – it will continue to confound you. The world will keep turning and changing. You will still need to make decisions and adjustments. It is best to remain flexible and apply to your daily life the self-awareness, the congruence and the discipline that have served you in good stead for years and years.

One day you'll realise there's no longer the need to fret about ageing. You are finally and undeniably old. Congruence should make you consider this a blessing. You've had your share of victories – well-received projects, jobs well done, happy associations. You have survived heartaches, illnesses, betrayals and failed dreams. On balance your life has been a good one.

• Of course you are still entitled to have dreams. And this is the beautiful part of being old – dreams are no longer aspirations accompanied with the fever of acquisitiveness. They are pleasurable images that float about – sitting in a cottage by the sea, walking through a field of wildflowers, listening to a choir in a medieval cathedral and laughing with children. They become part of your reflections. They soothe you. They are part of a new reality where you stand on the precipice of the last undefined adventure. You don't know exactly when you'll be made to take the plunge. What does it matter? You've reached this far where you can examine life from various vantage points. It's a feat that's not granted to everyone. Be thankful.

NOTES

NOTES